Competency-based Practical Manual of PHARMACOLOGY

Competency-based Practical Manual of
PHARMACOLOGY

As per the Revised Competency-based Medical Education Curriculum (NMC)

SECOND EDITION

Apurva Agrawal MBBS MD (Pharmacology) MAMS ACME
Professor
Department of Pharmacology
RNT Medical College
Udaipur, Rajasthan, India

Harcharan Singh MBBS MD (Pharmacology)
Professor
Department of Pharmacology
RNT Medical College
Udaipur, Rajasthan, India

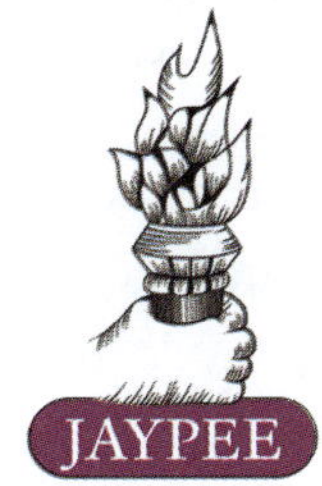

JAYPEE BROTHERS MEDICAL PUBLISHERS
The Health Sciences Publisher
New Delhi | London

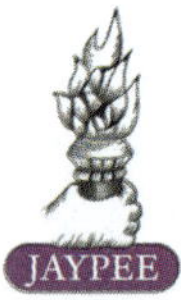

Jaypee Brothers Medical Publishers (P) Ltd

Headquarters
EMCA House
23/23-B, Ansari Road, Daryaganj
New Delhi 110 002, India
Landline: +91-11-23272143, +91-11-23272703
+91-11-23282021, +91-11-23245672
E-mail: jaypee@jaypeebrothers.com

Corporate Office
4838/24, Ansari Road, Daryaganj
New Delhi 110 002, India
Phone: +91-11-43574357
Fax: +91-11-43574314
E-mail: jaypee@jaypeebrothers.com

Overseas Office
J.P. Medical Ltd
83 Victoria Street, London
SW1H 0HW (UK)
Phone: +44 20 3170 8910
E-mail: info@jpmedpub.com

EU GPSR Authorised Representative
Logos Europe, 9 rue Nicolas Poussin
17000, La Rochelle, France
Phone: +33 (0) 6 67 93 73 78
E-mail: contact@logoseurope.eu

Website: www.jaypeebrothers.com
Website: www.jaypeedigital.com

Competency-based Practical Manual of Pharmacology

First Edition: 2023

Second Edition: **2026**

ISBN: 978-93-6616-496-0

Printed in India at Sterling Graphics Pvt. Ltd.

Certificate

This is certified that .... of Second Professional MBBS has satisfactorily completed all the competencies in Clinical and Applied Pharmacology. It is certified that he/she has satisfactorily completed required number of procedures in the certifiable competencies.

Date: ....

Place: ....

Signature and Seal
Head of Department

Preface to the Second Edition

Pharmacology is a dynamic subject which needs continuous updating as new drugs are being added to the armor, as well as with the evolution of new evidence, treatment regimens also keep on changing. As per National Medical Council's (NMC's) recent competency-based medical education (CBME) curriculum guidelines 2024, at the end of the second professional year of MBBS, a student should be able to not only understand various drugs but also rationally prescribe them, identify and manage adverse drug reactions, and communicate with the patients regarding medicines and their uses. In the 2nd edition, four new chapters have been added according to modifications in the NMC guidelines. The new chapters include one chapter on sources of drug information and three chapters on attitude, ethics, and communication (AETCOM) modules that have to be taught by the pharmacology faculty. Other chapters have also been revised according to modifications in the competencies. This 2nd edition of manual is an effort to provide authentic resource material covering all competencies suggested by the latest NMC guidelines for practical and small group learning in Pharmacology.

Apurva Agrawal

Harcharan Singh

Preface to the First Edition

Pharmacology deals with each and every aspect of drugs. One of the main goals of teaching pharmacology to second professional MBBS students is to inculcate the basic principles of rational prescribing right from the beginning. With the implementation of competency-based medical education (CBME) in 2019, practical teaching in Pharmacology has significantly changed. The details of pharmacy preparations and animal experiment based exercises which were previously taught have now been limited. The new curriculum has included competencies related to dosage forms, drug delivery devices, pharmacovigilance, prescription writing, prescription audit, P-drug list, essential medicine list, drug promotional literature, drug interactions and dose calculations. Animal experiments are now replaced by computer assisted learning (CAL) based simulation exercises. Communication skills have been given special emphasis, and many competencies have been added regarding communication with patients, peers and pharmaceutical representatives. This huge change needed a modification in the practical teaching methods and the practical manual. This practical manual is an effort to provide an authentic resource material covering all the competencies suggested by National Medical Council (NMC) for practical and small group learning in Pharmacology.

Apurva Agrawal

Harcharan Singh

Acknowledgments

Learning is a lifelong process and, in this journey, we meet many teachers who inspire us. We acknowledge all our teachers and seniors who have been instrumental in our learning and understanding of Pharmacology. We are grateful to all faculty members of the Department of Pharmacology, RNT Medical College, Udaipur, Rajasthan, India, for having faith in us. We acknowledge all the students and their quest for learning, which has encouraged us to write this manual. We acknowledge the resident doctors of the department who have been immensely helpful in proofreading and editing work. We are deeply indebted to our parents and family for supporting us wholeheartedly in all our endeavors. Lastly, we would like to thank our publisher M/s Jaypee Brothers Medical Publishers (P) Ltd, New Delhi, India, for entrusting confidence in us.

Competency Terminologies

Competency

It is an observable ability that a medical student is required to acquire, integrating multiple components such as knowledge, skills, values and attitude.

Domain

It is the area of specialization(s) for a specific competency. Four domains has been advised by NMC, and a competency can address a single or a mix of two or more domains.

- K—Knowledge
- S—Skill
- A—Attitude
- C—Communication

Level of Competency

It defines the level that a medical student is able to achieve, in order to acquire a specific competency. It is based on the Miller's pyramid.

- K—Knows
- KH—Knows How
- S—Shows
- SH—Shows How
- P—Performs Individually

Core

It defines whether the competency belongs to a 'core' area or a 'desirable' one.

- Y—Yes, core
- N—Non-core

Teaching Learning (TL) Methods

Various teaching learning methods have been advised by NMC for a specific competency depending on the domain and level of competency.

- Lecture
- Small group discussion
- Bedside clinic
- DOAP (Demonstrate, Observe, Assist, Perform)
- Practical session
- Skill station
- Skill lab

Assessment Method

National Medical Council (NMC) has also suggested the assessment method for every competency depending on the domain(s) it is covering and the level of competency.

- Written
- Viva voce

- Skill assessment
- Skill station
- Maintenance of Logbook
- Objective Structured Clinical Examination (OSCE)/Objective Structured Practical Examination (OSPE)

Certification (P)

For some competencies it is mandatory to certify that a student was able to perform that particular skill independently, a number (P) of times.

Contents

* Certifiable Competencies (Total 11 competencies are certifiable)

CHAPTER 1

Drug Nomenclature

COMPETENCY

PH1.3: Describe nomenclature of drugs.

DRUG

- It is derived from a French word "Drogue" meaning "a dry herb". WHO defines drug as "any substance or product that is used or intended to be used, to modify or explore, physiological systems or pathological states for the benefit of the recipient".
- 'Medicine' term is more frequently used as the term 'Drug' also refers to psychoactive substances.
- **Psychoactive drugs**: These are substances which, when taken in or administered into one's system, affect mental processes, e.g., perception, consciousness, cognition or mood and emotions.
- A drug could have chemical name, International nonproprietary name (INN) or brand name.

Chemical Name

Chemical name describes the chemical structure/character of drug. It is given by International Union of Pure and Applied Chemistry (IUPAC). These names are complex and difficult to remember for day-to-day practice, e.g., N-Acetyl-p-aminophenol (Paracetamol).

International Nonproprietary Name

- The name that is accepted by competent authority at National/International level is known as nonproprietary name, e.g., propranolol. INN is given to any substance by INN Expert Group on the request of WHO. The INN system simplifies the nomenclature of drugs and incorporates uniformity. These names are recognized all over the globe by all countries and do not vary with the manufacturing company.
- There could be British Approved Name (BAN) or United States Approved Name (USAN).
- Some old names are accepted as such due to their popularity, e.g., aspirin.
- Paracetamol, Salbutamol and Adrenaline are BAN, which are known as Acetaminophen, Albuterol and Epinephrine respectively by USAN

Note: Nonproprietary names are also called as 'Generic Name', but this term is a misnomer. It is better to use the term 'Nonproprietary name'.

Proprietary Name/Trade Name/Brand Name

This name is given by the manufacturer. All drugs are available in the market by their brand name. Brand names are catchy, easier to remember and propagated by pharmaceutical companies. On the other hand, brand names of a single medicine vary with different manufacturers. Even the same manufacturer might sell the same drug by different names in different geographical areas. This creates confusion and sometime might result in medication errors.

Pharmacopeias

Pharmacopeias are official publications by competent authorities that contain information regarding chemical structure, molecular weight, physical characteristics, chemical characteristics, identification methods, assays, purity standards, standards for storage and dosage forms of drugs approved in that country.

- **IP:** Indian Pharmacopeia
- **BP:** British Pharmacopeia
- **USP:** United States Pharmacopeia

Drug Formulary

Formularies include information related to dose, dosage forms available, indications, precautions and adverse effects of drugs available in a country. They are useful for medical practitioners. A hospital could also have a drug formulary of drugs available in their pharmacy.

- **NFI:** National Formulary of India
- **BNF:** British National Formulary

Orphan Drugs

Drugs meant for diagnosis, treatment or prevention of rare diseases or for conditions, for which the cost of developing and marketing is not expected to be recovered from sales, are termed as orphan drugs. Tax benefits or other incentives are offered by Government for development and production of orphan drugs.

Essential Drugs

These are the drugs that satisfy the healthcare needs of the population. These drugs are selected on the basis of public health relevance, evidence of efficacy, safety and cost effectiveness. They should be available at all times, in appropriate dosage forms, appropriate quality, adequate amount, with appropriate information, at a cost that is affordable by an individual and community, and within the context of functioning health system.

Over the Counter (OTC) Drugs

Drugs that are generally considered safe and are meant for common ailments, could be directly purchased from pharmacy stores without the need of Doctor's prescription, are known as OTC drugs, e.g., paracetamol, ibuprofen, antacids, laxatives, etc.

Prescription Only Drugs (Schedule H Drugs)

Drugs that could be dispensed by any pharmacy store only when prescribed by a registered medical practitioner are known as prescription-only drugs, e.g., antibiotics. Tablet packs with red strip indicate that particular medicine is a prescription-only drug.

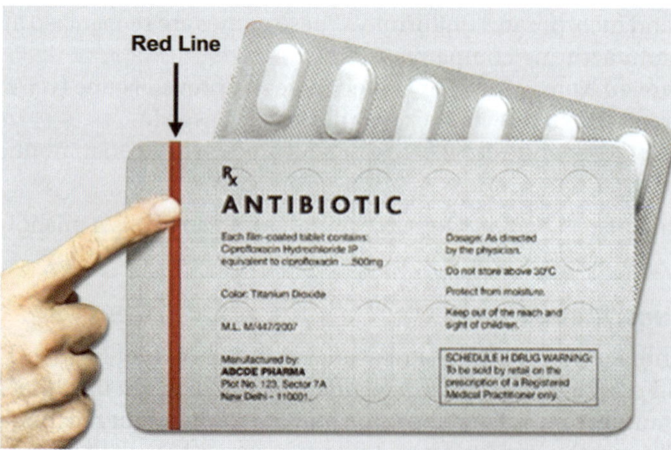

Schedule X Drugs

Drugs included in this category are psychotropic drugs. They are also prescription only drugs. Pharmacy stores need a license to keep these drugs. They should be kept under lock and key, and the pharmacist must retain the copy of prescription for at least two years, e.g., amphetamine, ketamine, etc.

Schedule G Drugs

These drugs can be given only under supervision of a registered medical practitioner. The drug label displays 'Caution: it is dangerous to take this preparation except under medical supervision.' Example: Bleomycin, busulphan, diphenhydramine.

Other Important Definitions

Expiry Date

This date reflects the duration up to which the product is known to remain stable in terms of strength, quality and purity. It is indicated that drugs should not be consumed after their expiry dates. But majority of drugs still retain their potency even after five years of their expiry date. Solid oral dosage forms, e.g., tablets and capsules, are most stable after expiry date is passed. Drugs in solution dosage form or as a reconstituted suspension may not have same potency if used outdated. So, in true sense expiry date is that date up to which the manufacturer can guarantee full potency and safety of that drug.

Shelf-life

The time period during which a drug product retains its potency if stored in specified conditions. Shelf-life is generally much longer than the expiry date.

EXERCISES

Exercise 1: Enumerate the advantages and disadvantages of prescribing drugs by their proprietary name.

Exercise 2: Enumerate the advantages and disadvantages of prescribing drugs by their nonproprietary name.

Exercise 3: What is the importance of expiry date of any drug product?

Exercise 4: Separate proprietary and nonproprietary names

Proprietary name | Nonproprietary name

1. Calpol, Paracetamol
2. Inderal, Propranolol
3. Ibuprofen, Combiflame
4. Oflox, Ofloxacin
5. Enalapril maleate, Envas

Exercise 5: Identify the different components of a DRUG LABEL. Enumerate them with significance of each.

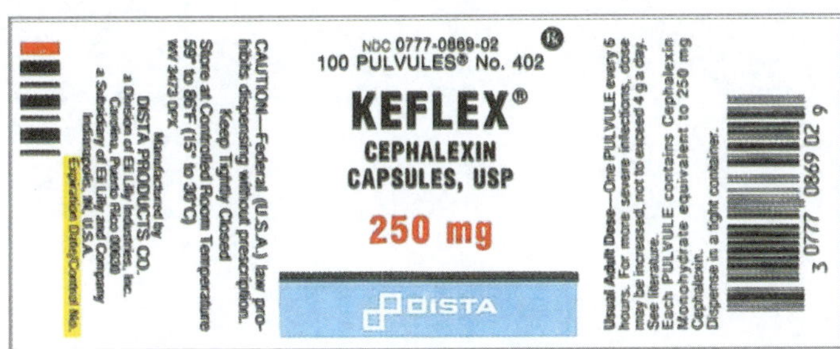

NOTES

CHAPTER

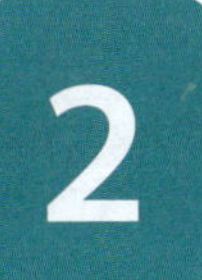

2

Sources of Drug Information

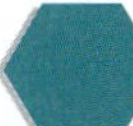

COMPETENCY

PH10.1: Compare and contrast different sources of drug information and update on latest information on drugs.

INTRODUCTION

Selection of the right drug for a disease, in a patient, must be supported by reliable, comprehensive and objective information about the drug. Extensive literature is available online that is also easy to access, but it raises concerns regarding the credibility and appropriateness of the information. In today's era of unlimited sources of information, it is important to identify reliable sources of drug information.

SOURCES OF DRUG INFORMATION

The sources of drug information are classified into three categories:

1. Primary sources
2. Secondary sources
3. Tertiary sources

Primary Sources of Drug Information

Primary sources include original research articles published in scientific journals and clinical drug trial reports. They provide information in the form of factual data. Here it is important to understand that all published articles in a journal are not considered primary sources, e.g., editorials and review articles are not considered primary sources of information.

Secondary Sources of Drug Information

Secondary sources are derived from primary sources of information. They include review articles, systematic reviews and meta-analyses. Abstracting or indexing services that compile published articles are also considered secondary sources of information as they direct a user to the relevant primary literature. Examples include Medline, PubMed, Index Medicus and Excerpta Medica.

Tertiary Sources of Drug Information

Tertiary sources include documents that are written by subject experts. Tertiary literature provides information that has been summarized and is often peer-reviewed. It includes textbooks, reference books, formularies, treatment guidelines, the National List of Essential Medicines (NLEM), etc.

Note: Review articles published in journals are regarded as secondary sources by some experts and tertiary sources of information by others.

Ideally one should first refer to tertiary source, then to secondary source and then to primary source of drug information.

Some Reliable Tertiary Sources of Drug Information

- **Pharmacopeia:** It is an official publications by competent authorities that contain information regarding chemical structure, molecular weight, physical characteristics, chemical characteristics, identification methods, assays, purity standards, standards for storage and dosage forms of drugs approved in that country.
  As per drug regulatory authority Pharmacopeia has legal standing in its country.
  - *IP:* Indian Pharmacopeia
  - *BP:* British Pharmacopeia
  - *USP:* United States Pharmacopeia
- **Drug formulary:** Formularies include information related to dose, dosage forms available, indications, precautions and adverse effects of drugs available in a country. A hospital could also have a drug formulary of drugs available in their pharmacy.
  They are useful for medical practitioners and provide up-to-date guidance to the prescribers.
  - *NFI:* National Formulary of India
  - *BNF:* British National Formulary
- **Martindale: The complete drug reference**—it is a compendium published by the Royal Pharmaceutical Society of Great Britain. It provides unbiased information on drugs used around the world. It also includes information on pharmaceutical excipients, radiopharmaceuticals, diagnostic agents, plant drugs, toxins and poisons.

COMMERCIAL PUBLICATIONS

Some commercial publications are also available that provide information regarding brands of medicines, formulations, cost, dose, adverse effects, precautions, contraindications, etc. Examples include Physician's Desk Reference, Indian Drug Review (IDR), Monthly Index of Medical Specialities (MIMS), etc.

UNRELIABLE SOURCES OF DRUG INFORMATION

- Friends, family members, television, magazines, drug advertisements and unauthorized online sites are considered unreliable sources of information.
- Drug Promotional Literature (DPL) provided by pharmaceutical representatives should always be checked for correctness and completeness. Sometimes they might contain incomplete and biased information.

EXERCISES

Exercise 1: Describe the differences between primary, secondary and tertiary sources of drug information.

Exercise 2: A second professional-year medical student wants to acquire information regarding the role of beta blockers in congestive heart failure. He should look for this information from which type of literature and why.

Exercise 3: A research scholar is planning to conduct a study on the comparative efficacy of celiprolol and nebivolol on blood pressure control. She should consult which type of literature while planning her research and why.

NOTES

CHAPTER 3

Solid Dosage Forms

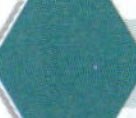

COMPETENCIES

PH1.4: Identify the common drug formulations and drug delivery systems, demonstrate their use and describe their advantages and disadvantages.
PH1.5: Describe various routes of drug administration, their advantages and disadvantages and demonstrate administration.

DOSAGE FORM

Dosage form is the physical form in which any drug is available for administration.

DRUG FORMULATION

It is the process by which a number of substances are combined with the active medication to finally produce a drug product that can be successfully given to patients. Apart from active ingredient(s), a drug formulation also contains excipients like diluents, preservatives, vehicles, etc.

ORAL SOLID DOSAGE FORMS

Tablets

In this dosage form the active ingredient (medicine) is mixed with binding agents, excipients, coloring agents, etc., and compressed into small oval or discoid shapes that are suitable for swallowing.

Tablets can be classified in different ways:

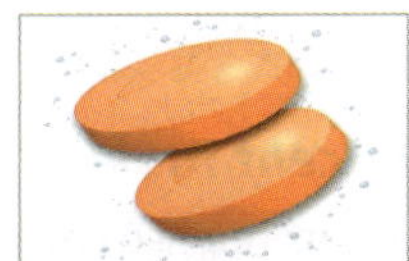

Uncoated tablets

Uncoated Tablets

Tablets without any specific coating are termed uncoated tablets.

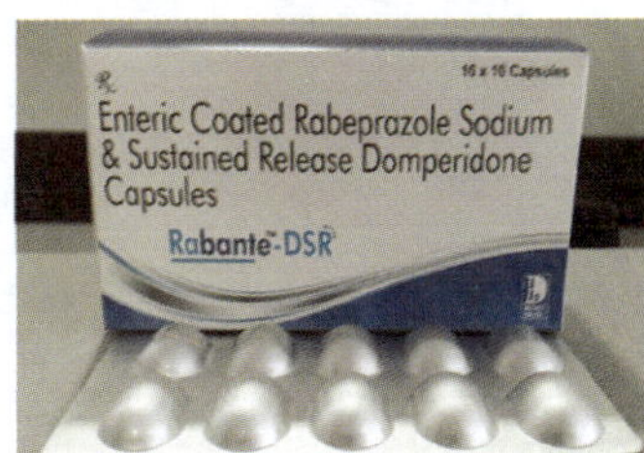

Enteric coated tablets

Coated Tablets

These are having a coating over them, e.g., sugar coated, enteric coated. Coated tablets must be swallowed completely without breaking or chewing them. If the coating is broken advantage of coated tablet is lost.

- **Sugar-coated tablets**: Sugar coating improves palatability. They are sweet in taste and preferred in children. Some bitter drugs are also available as sugar coated tablet, e.g., chloroquine.
- **Enteric coated tablet**: Tablet is coated with a material that does not allow release of drug in acidic pH of the stomach thereby protecting the drug that could be destroyed by gastric juices. The drug is released only when it reaches in the alkaline medium of small intestine. This should be swallowed as a whole without chewing or breaking.

Scored Tablet and Unscored Tablet

- Scored tablet is provided with a groove or 'score line' that divides the tablet into 2 or 4 equal parts. This helps in breaking the tablet into equal parts. It provides dose flexibility and ease of swallowing.
- Tablets without any such score line are termed as unscored tablets.

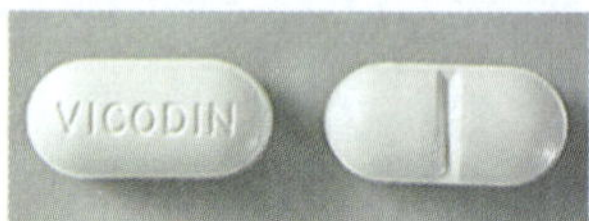

Scored tablets

Immediate Release (IR) Tablets

They dissolve and release active ingredient immediately in the stomach. Most of the tablets are IR tablet unless mentioned otherwise.

Sustained/Extended-release Tablets

The drug particles are coated in such a way that they are released at different rates. This dosage form prolong the duration of action of short acting drugs. This reduces frequency of drug administration and improves patient compliance. It must be swallowed as a whole. It contains higher dose meant to act for long time. If it is broken and coating is disturbed, there is a risk of exposure to large doses and toxicity.

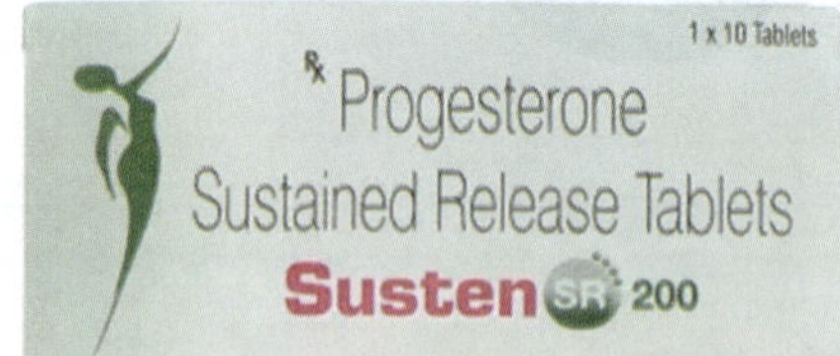

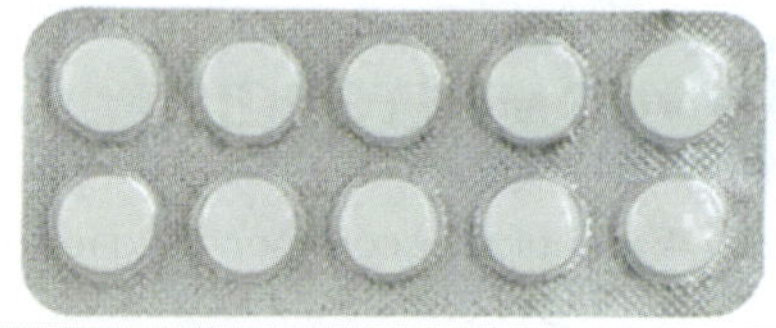
Sustained/extended-release tablets

Controlled Release Tablet

It contains a semipermeable membrane that controls the release of drug and makes it long acting. This also must be swallowed as a whole.

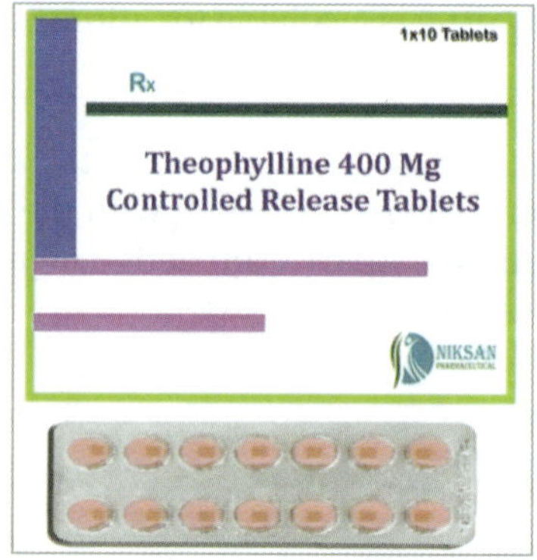

Controlled release tablet

Effervescent Tablet

Such tablets release carbon dioxide when they come in contact with water. This helps in quick disintegration and dissolution in water. It improves palatability and imparts a psychological effect on patients.

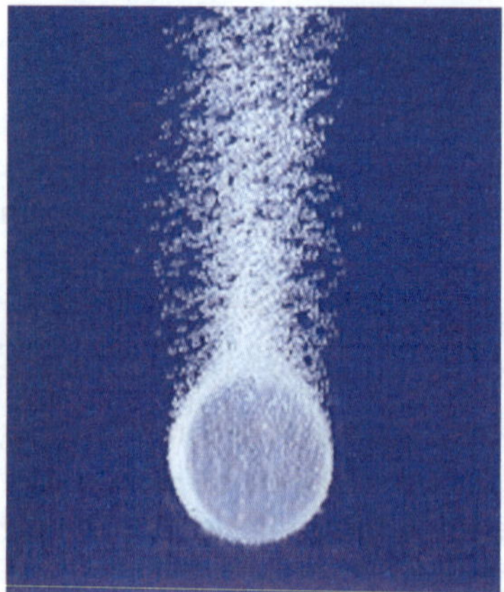
Effervescent tablet

Dispersible Tablet

It is added to a small amount of water in which it disperses quickly. This improves the rate of absorption. Example: Dispersible tablet of aspirin.

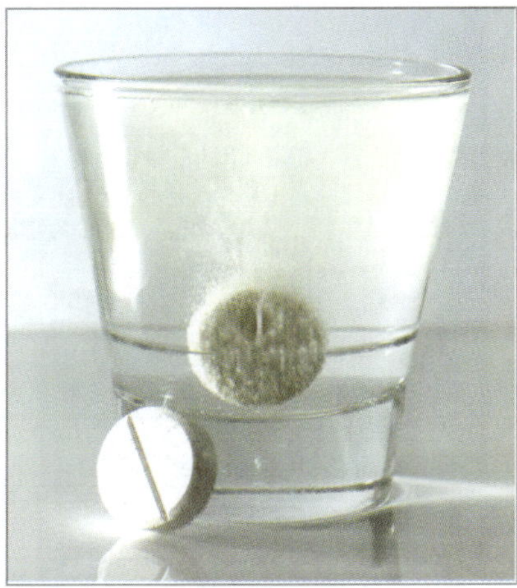

Dispersible tablet

Sublingual Tablet

This tablet when placed beneath the tongue, it disintegrates and dissolves rapidly and gets immediately absorbed, bypassing the gastrointestinal tract (GIT) and first pass metabolism. Rapid onset, higher bioavailability and rapid termination on spitting are its advantages. Example: Nitroglycerine

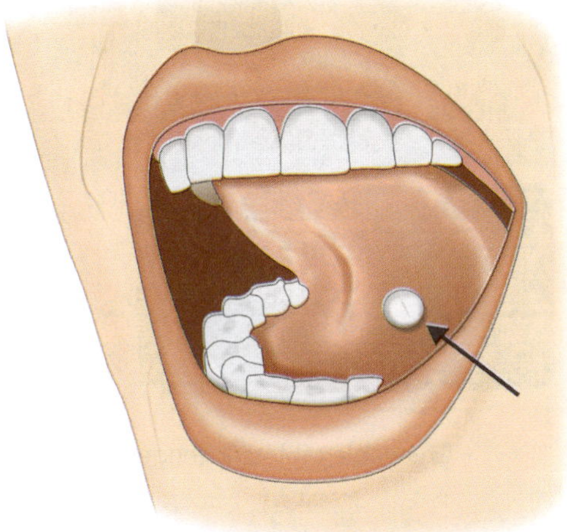

Sublingual tablet

Capsule

In this dosage form, powdered or liquid drug is contained in water soluble cylindrical containers made of gelatin. Capsules usually have better patient compliance due to bland taste.

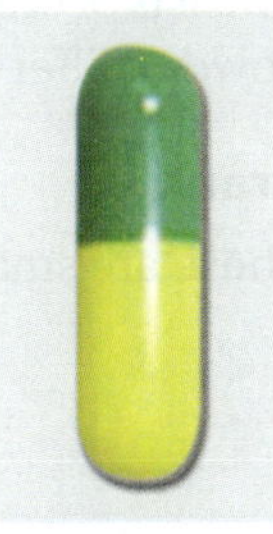

Hard capsule

Types of capsules:

Hard Capsule

It is a two-piece cylindrical structure that may contain medicine in the form of powder or liquid. The powdered medicine could be manually filled and prepared when required for research purposes.

Soft Capsule

It is one piece gelatin capsule containing liquid or semi-solid medicine. Oily medicines could be easily administered using this dosage form.

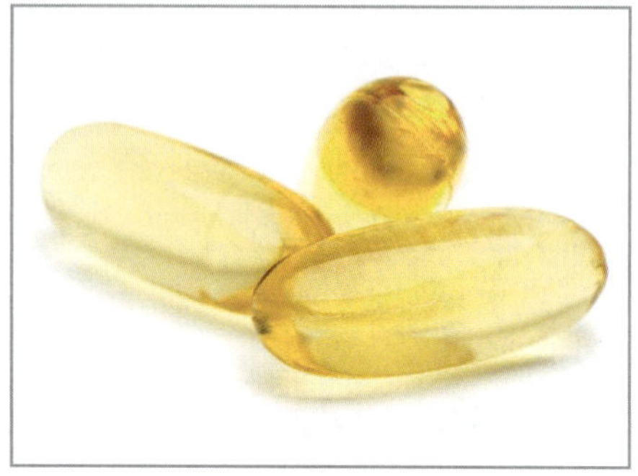

Soft capsule

Spansules

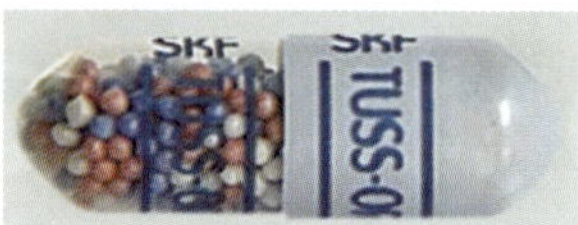

Spansules

It consists of variable coating that releases the medicament gradually in a time based manner. It is also known as timesule.

Chewable Tablet/Lozenges

This solid dosage form contain drug along with a suitable gum, sweetening and flavoring agent. It is meant to be kept in mouth and not to be swallowed. Lozenges act by increasing salivary secretion and soothe local mucosa in mouth and throat.

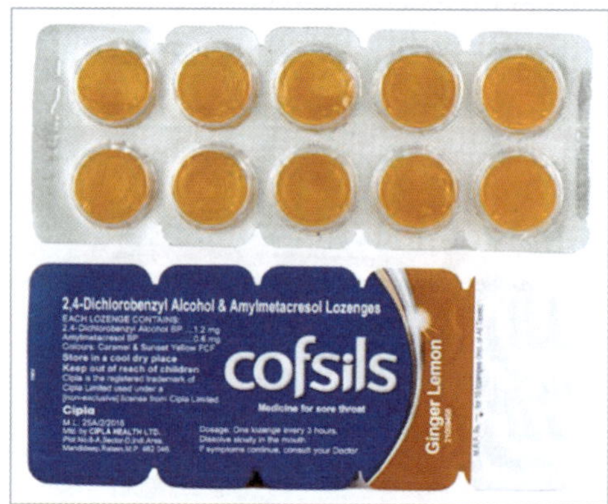

Chewable tablets/lozenges

Powders

The drug is available in finely divided solid form. Powders could be simple powder and compound powder. Simple powder consists of only single medicament, e.g., glucose powder. Compound powder consists of multiple medicaments, e.g., ORS powder. Effervescent powder is also available that releases carbon dioxide when combined with water, e.g., Eno powder.

Granules

These are small aggregates of powder held together by binding agents, e.g., vitamin D granules.

SOLID TOPICAL DOSAGE FORMS

Dusting Powder

The drug is in the form of finely divided particles meant for external use, e.g., neosporin powder

Plasters

These are solid adhesive preparations applied to protect and provide mechanical support to underlying body area, e.g., plaster of Paris.

OTHER SOLID DOSAGE FORMS

Suppository

It is a solid dosage form that is inserted in the body through rectum, vagina or urethra, to slowly release the medicine. They are conical at one end for ease of insertion and made up of a substance that melts at body temperature, e.g., cocoa butter, carbowax. Suppositories for vagina are known as pessaries while those for urethra are known as bougies.

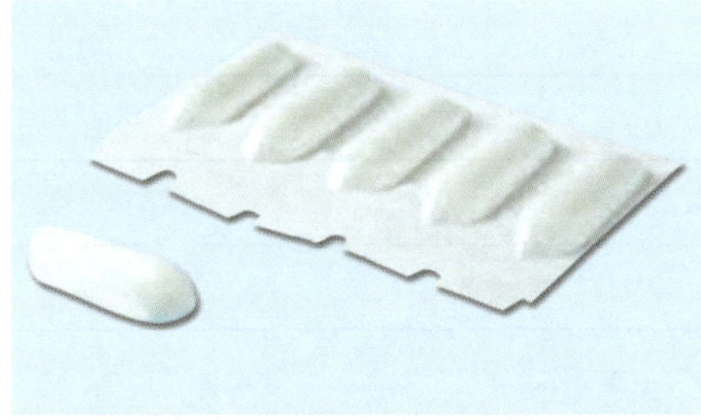

Suppository

Guidelines for self-administration of rectal suppository:

1. Wash your hands.
2. Remove the covering.
3. If the suppository is too soft let it harden first by cooling it (fridge or hold under cold running water, still packed!) then remove covering.
4. Remove any possible sharp rims by warming in the hand.
5. Moisten the suppository with cold water.
6. Lie on your side and pull up your knees.
7. Gently insert the suppository, conical end first, into the anal passage.
8. Remain lying down for several minutes.
9. Wash your hands.
10. Try not to have a bowel movement during the first hour.

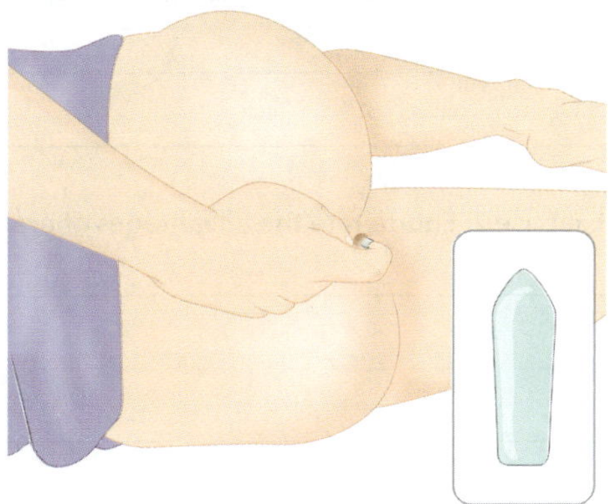

Rectal suppository

Pellets

These are sterile solid structures made by compression of drug, implanted subcutaneously as depot preparation. The drug is slowly released from the preparation, e.g., testosterone.

Transdermal Patch

It is an adhesive device to be applied on the skin that delivers the drug at a constant rate for systemic absorption. The drug is contained in a reservoir between a backing film and a micropore membrane that controls the rate of drug delivery. Common sites of application are upper arm, chest, abdomen, lower back, etc.

Guidelines for self-administration of transdermal patch application:

1. For patch site, see the instructions provided with the drug or check with the pharmacist.
2. Do not apply over bruised or damaged skin.
3. Do not wear over skin folds or under tight clothing and change spots regularly.
4. Apply with clean, dry hands.
5. Clean and dry the area of application completely.
6. Remove the patch from the package, do not touch the 'drug' side.
7. Place on the skin and press firmly.
8. Rub the edges to seal.
9. Remove and replace according to instructions given.

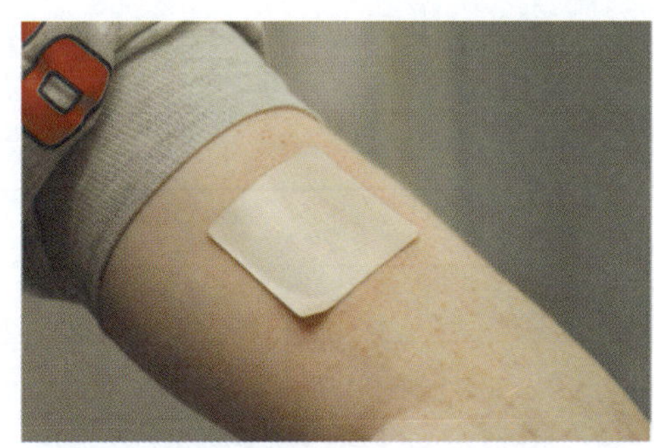

Transdermal patch

EXERCISES

Exercise 1: Mention any five oral solid dosage forms with one specific feature of each.

Exercise 2: Enumerate the advantages of oral solid dosage forms.

Exercise 3: Enumerate the disadvantages of oral solid dosage forms.

Exercise 4: What is the difference between sugar-coated and enteric-coated tablet?

Exercise 5: Enumerate the advantages of transdermal patch.

Exercise 6: Communicate with the patient in vernacular language on how to use a sublingual tablet.

NOTES

CHAPTER

Liquid and Semisolid Dosage Forms

COMPETENCIES

PH1.4: Identify the common drug formulations and drug delivery systems, demonstrate their use and describe their advantages and disadvantages.
PH1.5: Describe various routes of drug administration, their advantages and disadvantages and demonstrate administration.

LIQUID DOSAGE FORMS

These are liquid preparations meant for oral, topical or parenteral administration. In this chapter, liquid and semisolid dosage forms for oral and topical administration have been discussed.

Liquids oral formulations are easier to administer to children. They are better absorbed than solid formulations. Maintenance of liquid dosage forms is not easy. They are costlier than tablets and shelf-life is shorter than solid dosage forms.

ORAL LIQUID DOSAGE FORMS

Solution

Clear homogenous liquid preparations that contain one or more soluble chemical substances dissolved in a suitable solvent or a mixture of soluble solvents. They are not required to be shaken before use.

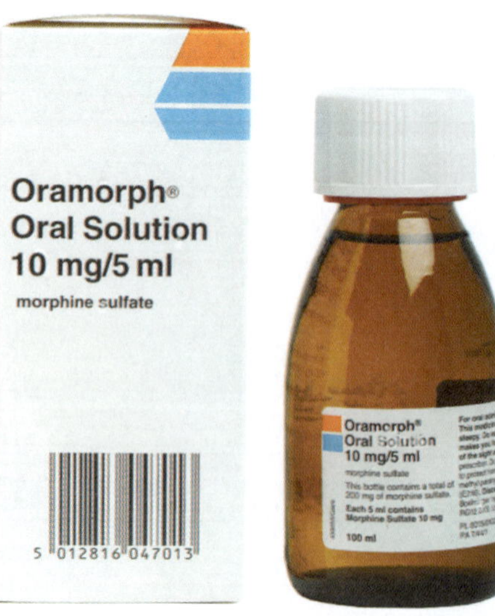

Solution

Suspension

A liquid medicament containing insoluble solid substances that are dispersed in water with the help of suspending agents. Specific instruction required is "SHAKE WELL BEFORE USE".

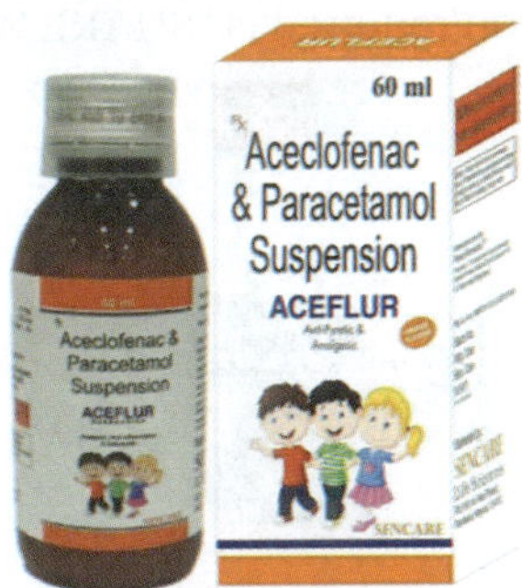

Suspension

Syrup

A liquid oral preparation in which concentrated aqueous solution of sucrose or other sugar is used as vehicle. They are sweet, thus mask unpleasant taste and are preferred in pediatric patients. For pediatric use syrups and suspensions are available in different flavors. It is important to keep them out of reach of children as there is a risk of poisoning, e.g., paracetamol poisoning.

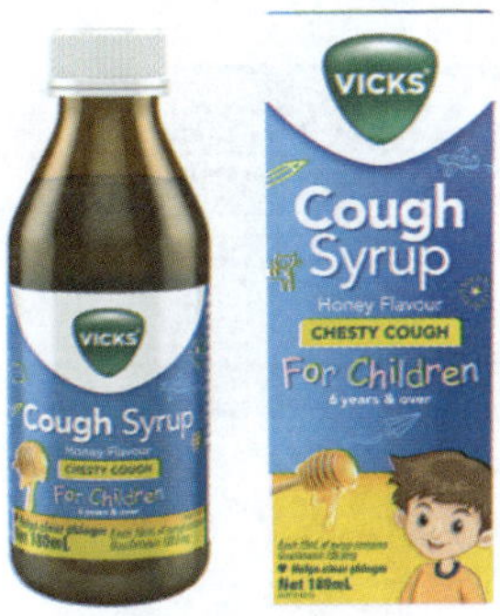

Syrup

Elixir

A clear liquid oral preparation that contains hydroalcoholic vehicle and has pleasant and sweet flavor. Elixirs are less viscous than syrups.

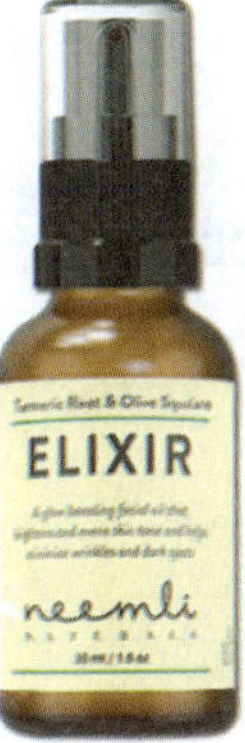

Elixir

Emulsion

A liquid medicament that contains two immiscible liquids. One of the two liquids is broken into small droplets (dispersed phase) and the other liquid surrounds each droplet as a film (continuous phase). Emulsions thus could be of two types, i.e., oil in water or water in oil. Specific instruction required is "SHAKE WELL BEFORE USE".

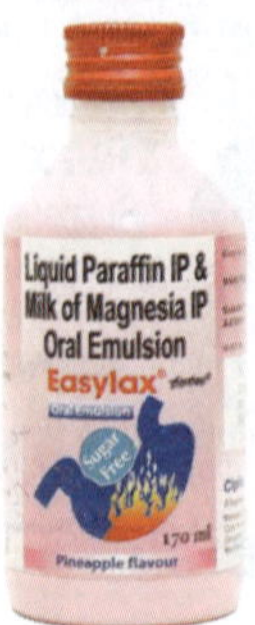

Emulsion

Mixtures

These are liquid dosage forms where soluble or insoluble solid drug particles are dispersed homogenously in a suitable vehicle. They are meant for internal use. If particles are insoluble, a suspending agent is added to keep them suspended, e.g., antidiarrheal mixture, milk of magnesia.

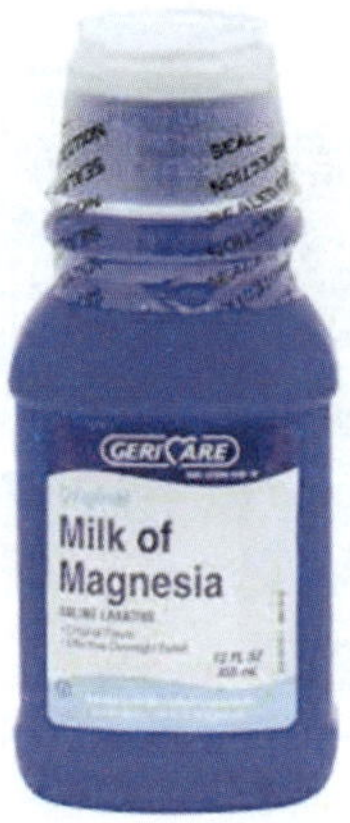

Mixtures

Drops

Liquid medicament that is administered by a dropper, meant for oral, nasal administration or topical administration in eye or ear canal. Oral drops are preferred in infants and young children due to ease of administration. Accurate dosing is possible by drops.

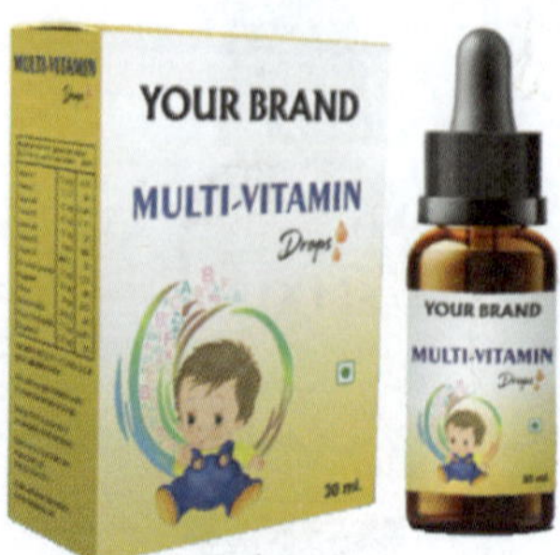

Drops

Guidelines for Self-administration of Eye Drops

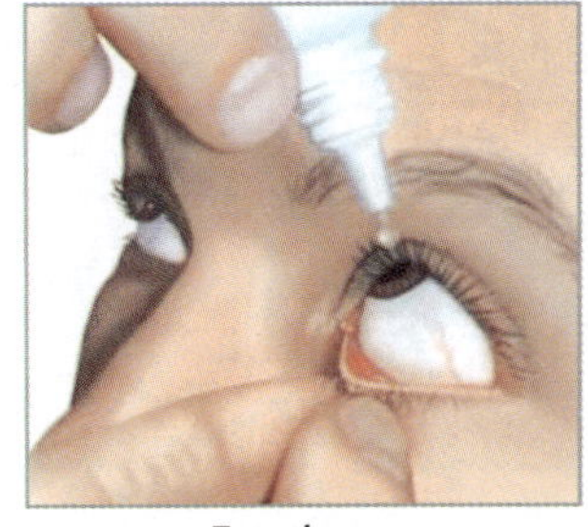
Eye drops

1. Wash your hands.
2. Do not touch the opening of the dropper.
3. Look upwards.
4. Pull the lower eyelid down to make a 'gutter'.
5. Bring the dropper as close to the 'gutter' as possible without touching it or the eye.
6. Apply the prescribed number of drops in the 'gutter'.
7. Close the eye for about two minutes but do not shut too tight.
8. If more than one kind of eye drop is used, wait at least for five minutes before applying the next drops.
9. Eye drops may cause a burning sensation but this should not last for more than a few minutes. If it does last longer, consult a doctor or pharmacist.

Guidelines for Self-administration of Ear Drops

1. Warm the ear-drops by rubbing them between the palms for several minutes, but do not use hot water.
2. Tilt the head sideways or lie on one side with the ear upward.
3. Gently pull the ear lobe to expose the ear canal.
4. Apply the number of drops prescribed.
5. Wait for five minutes before turning to the other ear.
6. Ear drops should not burn or sting for longer than a few minutes.

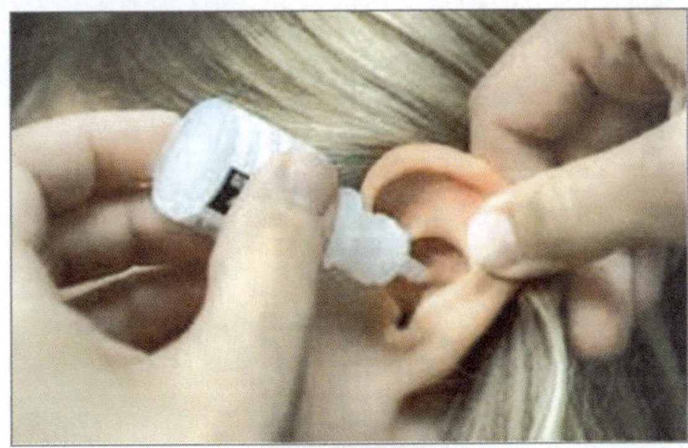
Ear drops

Guidelines for Self-administration of Nasal Drops

1. Blow the nose.
2. Sit down and tilt the head backwards completely or lie down with a pillow under the shoulders; keep head straight.
3. Insert the dropper approximately 1 cm into the nostril.
4. Apply the number of drops prescribed.
5. Immediately afterward, tilt the head forwards strongly (head between knees).
6. Sit up after a few seconds; the drops will then drip into the pharynx.
7. Repeat the procedure for the other nostril, if necessary.
8. Rinse the dropper with boiled water.

TOPICAL LIQUID AND SEMISOLID DOSAGE FORMS

Liquid and semisolid preparations are better for topical application than solid dosage forms, e.g., powders.

Lotion

A liquid preparation that is meant for external application on the skin and mucous membrane. It is applied without rubbing. It provides soothing, protective and emollient effects. Lotions are less viscous than creams and ointments, e.g., potassium permanganate lotion, calamine lotion.

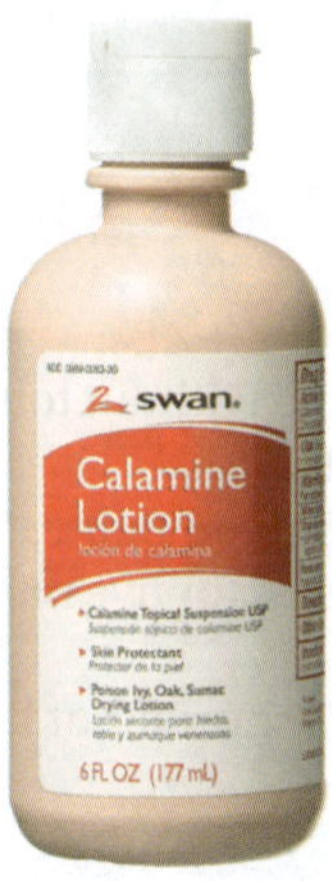

Lotion

Liniment

A liquid or semisolid preparation meant for external application on the skin. It is counterirritant in nature and is applied by rubbing on the skin. Its application may result in mild burning sensation and a feeling of warmth. Liniment should not be applied on broken skin or mucous membrane. It possesses analgesic and rubefacient properties, e.g., liniment turpentine, diclofenac liniment.

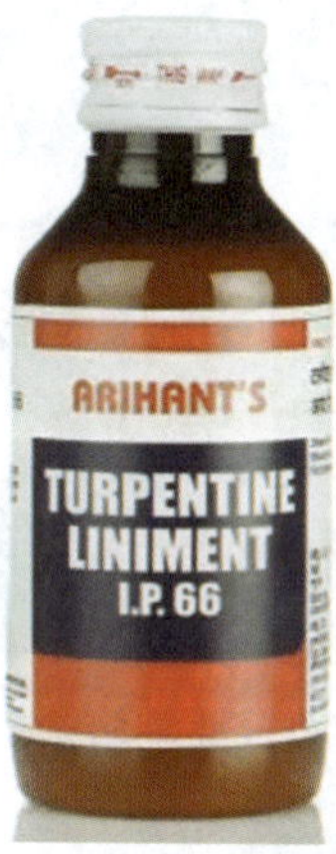

Liniment

Ointment

A semisolid preparation in greasy base that is meant for external application on the skin or mucous membrane. Ointments maintain the hydration of skin and stay for a long duration due to greasy nature. They may stain clothes and are less preferred by patients as compared to creams and lotions, e.g., Whitfield's ointment, antibiotic eye ointments.

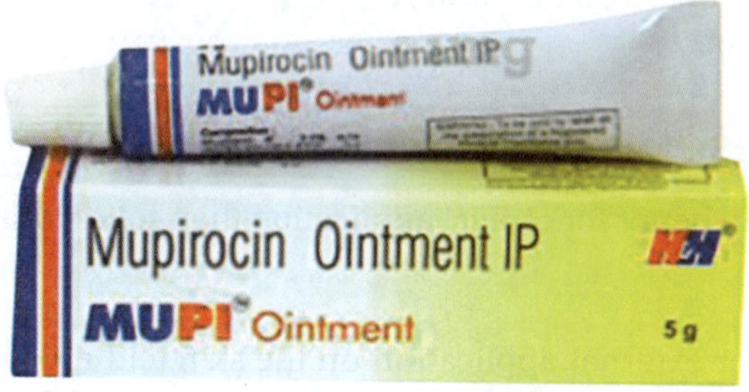

Ointment

Guidelines for Self-administration of Eye Ointment

1. Wash your hands.
2. Do not touch anything with the tip of the tube.
3. Tilt the head backwards a little.
4. Take the tube in one hand and pull down the lower eyelid with the other hand, to make a 'gutter'.
5. Bring the tip of the tube as close to the 'gutter' as possible.
6. Apply the amount of ointment prescribed.
7. Close the eye for two minutes.
8. Clean the tip of the tube with a tissue and recap the tube.

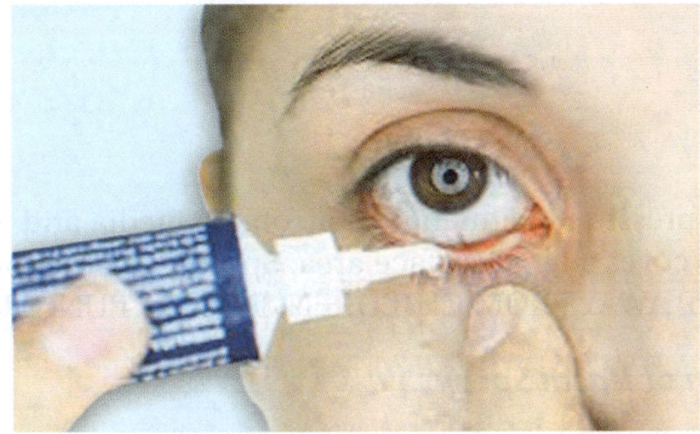

Eye ointment

Cream

A semisolid preparation containing oil in water emulsion and meant for external application on skin and mucous membrane. It is less greasy and is cosmetically better acceptable to patients. Creams are easily washed out and need multiple applications.

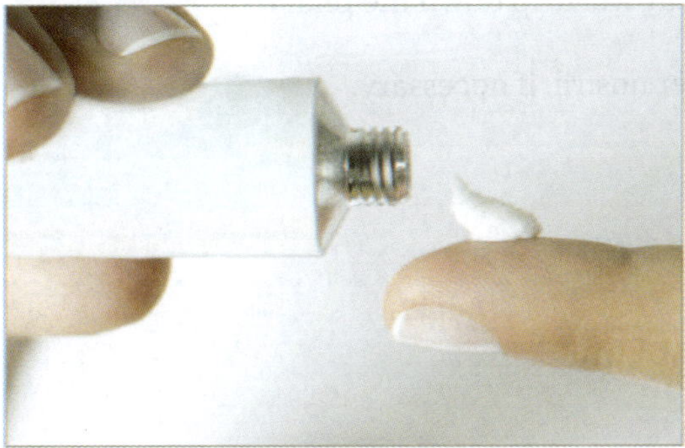

Cream

Gel

A viscous colloidal solution of gelatine containing medicament. It is meant for external application. Gels are less greasy than ointments.

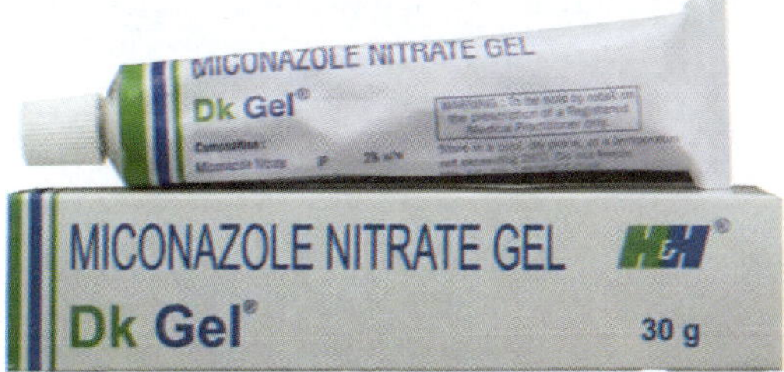

Gel

Paste

A semisolid dosage form of thick consistency containing hydrophilic powders like starch, chalk, zinc oxide, etc. It is non-greasy in nature. Toothpastes are used for dental hygiene.

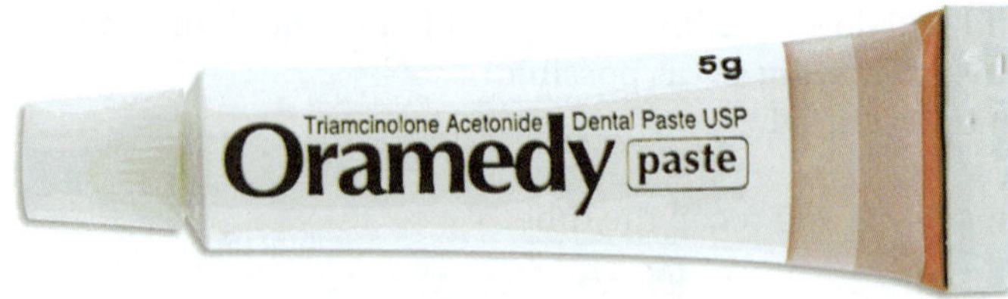

Paste

Spray

The medicament is packaged under pressure in aqueous or alcoholic media and is meant for application over skin or mucous membrane. Easy to use and cover a large surface area. Specific instructions required are: DO NOT SPRAY IN EYES, KEEP AWAY FROM HEAT, KEEP AWAY FROM CHILDREN, DO NOT PUNCTURE OR INCINERATE.

Guidelines for Self-administration of Nasal Spray

1. Blow the nose.
2. Sit with the head slightly tilted forward.
3. Shake the spray.
4. Insert the tip in one nostril.
5. Close the other nostril and mouth.
6. Spray by squeezing the vial (flask, container) and sniff slowly.
7. Remove the tip from the nose and bend the head forward strongly (head between the knees).
8. Sit up after a few seconds; the spray will drip down the pharynx.
9. Breathe through the mouth.
10. Repeat the procedure for the other nostril, if necessary.
11. Rinse the tip with boiled water.

EXERCISES

Exercise 1: Enumerate the advantages of oral liquid dosage forms.

Exercise 2: Enumerate the disadvantages of oral liquid dosage forms.

Exercise 3: Differentiate between a lotion and a liniment.

Exercise 4: Define solution, suspension and emulsion dosage forms. Mention specific instructions required with them.

Exercise 5: Write two advantages and disadvantages of ointment and cream dosage forms.

Exercise 6: Describe the counter-irritant mechanism of liniments.

Exercise 7: Communicate with the patient in vernacular language on how to correctly use eye drops.

NOTES

CHAPTER

Inhalational Dosage Forms

COMPETENCIES

PH1.4: Identify the common drug formulations and drug delivery systems, demonstrate their use and describe their advantages and disadvantages.
PH1.5: Describe various routes of drug administration, their advantages and disadvantages and demonstrate administration.

INTRODUCTION

Inhalational dosage forms enter the respiratory tract via the inhaled air and are thus termed inhalational dosage forms. Majority of them are meant to act at the respiratory tract for pulmonary diseases, e.g., inhalational drugs for treatment of asthma and chronic obstructive pulmonary disease (COPD). Some are meant for absorption in systemic circulation, e.g., anesthetic gases.

- **Aerosol:** These are very small solid particles or liquid droplets that are suspended in air or in a gas.
- **Dry powders**: These are available as finely divided particles and converted into aerosol through dry powder inhalers.
- **Gases**: These are mainly used for the purpose of general anesthesia, e.g., nitrous oxide, oxygen, etc.

To deliver inhalational dosage forms to the lungs, specialized delivery devices are required, e.g., metered dose inhaler, dry powder inhaler, rotahaler, and nebulizer.

METERED DOSE INHALER

Metered dose inhaler (MDI) is a small hand-held device for delivery of a metered dose of aerosol to the lungs. It contains a canister that is filled with pressurized medicine as solution or suspension of micronized drug particles dispersed in a suitable propellant.

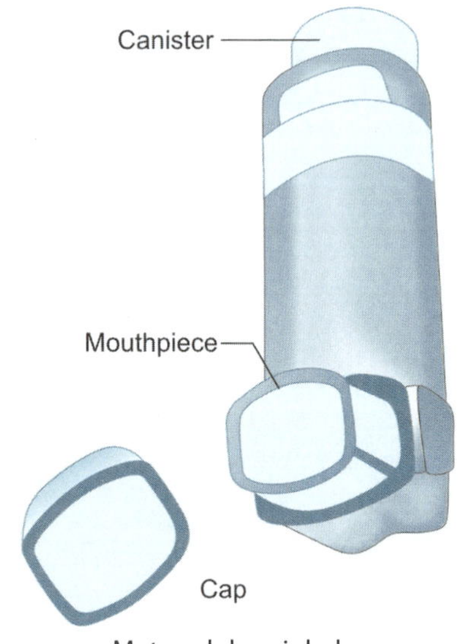

Metered dose inhaler

Steps for Self-administration of Metered Dose Inhaler/Aerosol

1. Cough up as much sputum as possible.
2. Shake the inhaler before use.
3. Hold the inhaler as indicated in the manufacturer's instructions (usually upside down).
4. Breathe out slowly, emptying the lungs of as much air as possible.
5. Place the lips tightly around the mouthpiece.
6. Tilt the head backward slightly.
7. Press the canister and breathe in deeply, keeping the tongue down.
8. Take the inhaler out and hold the breath for ten to fifteen seconds.
9. Breathe out slowly through the nose.
10. Rinse the mouth with warm water.

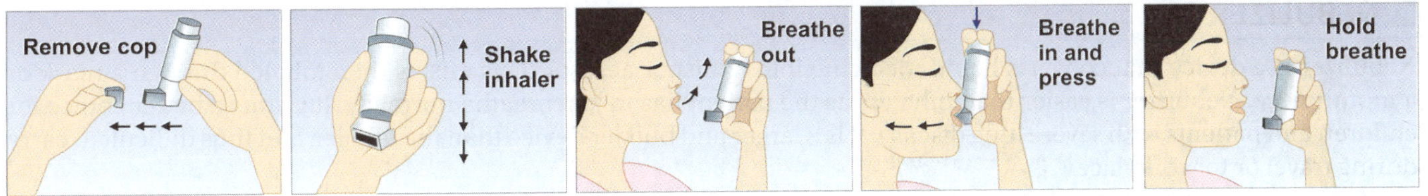

Steps for self-administration of metered dose inhaler (MDI)/aerosol

SPACER

Spacer is a device that introduces a space between the inhaler and patient's mouth. It is helpful in children as precise control is not required and the patient can simply breathe from the spacer. It is also indicated in patients taking steroid inhalation as larger particles get settled on the spacer's wall, thereby reducing the chances of swallowing and subsequent systemic as well as local adverse effects in the oral cavity.

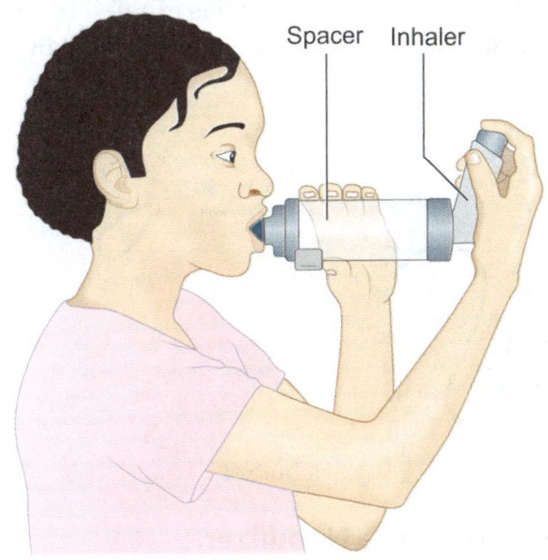

Spacer

DRY POWDER INHALER

In this device, drug is in the form of finely divided powder that is aerosolized by patient's own breath. If it is a capsule-based device then each time a capsule has to be inserted following the instructions of manufacturer. If it is a prefilled inhaler then a prefixed dose has to be released in the chamber following the instructions of manufacturer. In either of the above, inhale only after a click is heard. Rest all the steps are same.

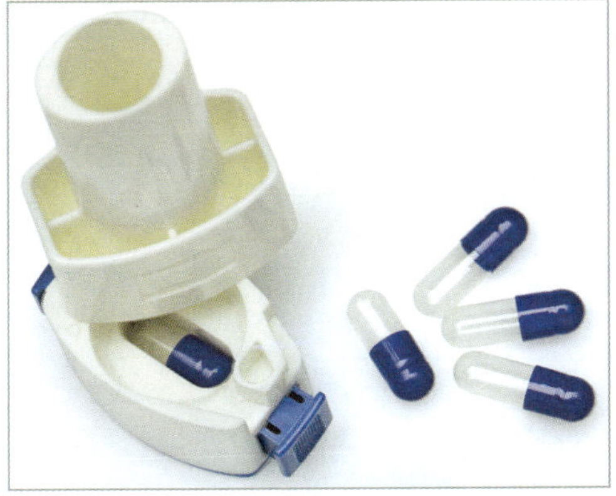

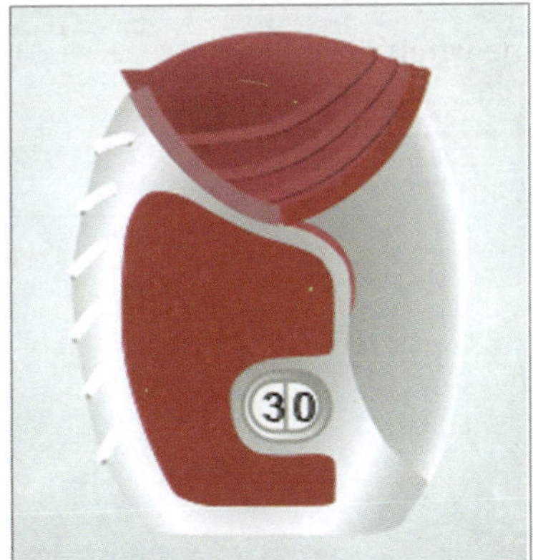

Dry powder inhaler

NEBULIZER

Nebulizer is a device that converts liquid medicine into a mist or aerosol. This mist is then inhaled through a mask or a mouthpiece. Nebulizer is easier than inhalers as the patient has to just breathe normally. It is thus a better choice for children and patients with severe lung disease. It is a larger and bulkier device than the inhaler, and thus difficult to carry during travel or to workplace.

Nebulizers are of following types:

- **Jet:** It uses compressed air to make aerosol.
- **Mesh:** In this liquid medicine passes through a fine mesh to produce aerosol.
- **Ultrasonic:** High frequency vibrations are used to produce aerosol.

A jet nebulizer contains the following parts:

- **Compressor:** It pumps outside air through the nozzle to the tubing.
- **Tubing:** It delivers compressed air from the compressor to the medication cup/nebulizing chamber.
- **Medication cup and Nebulizing chamber:** Liquid medication is poured in this cup which is then converted into aerosol
- **Face mask/mouthpiece:** The part through which the aerosol is inhaled by patient.
- **Nebulizer filter:** It helps to remove particulate matter in the compressed air.

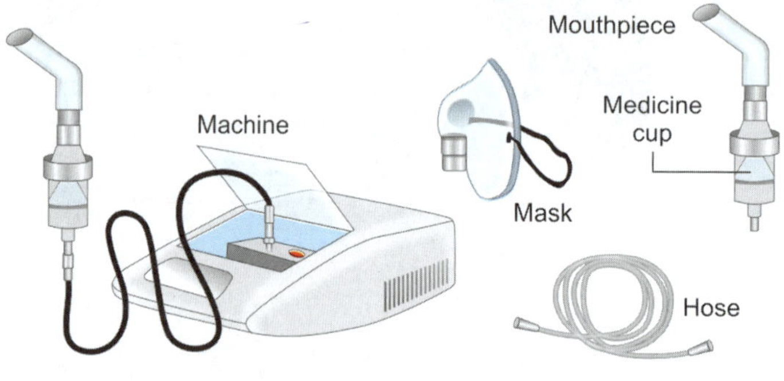

Nebulizer

Steps for Self-administration of Aerosol from a Nebulizer

- Wash your hands.
- Connect the tubing or hose to an air compressor.
- Fill the medicine cup with medicine, close the medicine cup tightly and always hold the mouthpiece straight up and down.
- Attach the other end of the hose to the mouthpiece and the medicine cup.
- Turn on the nebulizer machine.
- Place the mouthpiece in the mouth and keep your lips firmly around the mouthpiece so that all of the medicine goes into your lungs. If available, face mask is a better option for children.
- Breathe through your mouth until all the medicine is used. This may take 5–15 minutes, depending on the device and medicine used.
- Turn off the machine when done.

EXERCISES

Exercise 1: Mention the differences between MDI, DPI and nebulizer.

Exercise 2: Enumerate the advantages of inhalational route of drug administration.

Exercise 3: Enumerate the instructions required with use of steroid inhaler.

Exercise 4: Educate on a simulated patient in vernacular language 'how to use a MDI' by showing the steps of proper use of MDI.

NOTES

CHAPTER 6

Parenteral Dosage Forms and Delivery Devices

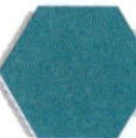

COMPETENCIES

PH1.4: Identify the common drug formulations and drug delivery systems, demonstrate their use and describe their advantages and disadvantages.
PH1.5: Describe various routes of drug administration, their advantages and disadvantages and demonstrate administration.

LIQUID DOSAGE FORMS FOR PARENTERAL ADMINISTRATION

For parenteral administration the liquid dosage forms are available as solutions, suspensions or emulsions.

- They must be sterile and pyrogen free.
- They should be clear and without any visible particulate matter.
- Any excipient used in them must be biocompatible.
- Many of them need to be maintained at specific temperature. This makes them costlier than dosage forms meant for oral administration.
- For parenteral administration some drugs are available in powder form with a suitable solvent that is added and a liquid preparation is formed just before administration.

For parenteral administration liquid dosage forms are dispensed in the following:

Ampoule

It is a small, sealed glass container containing sterile single time use medicine for parenteral administration. The neck of ampoule has to be broken to use it.

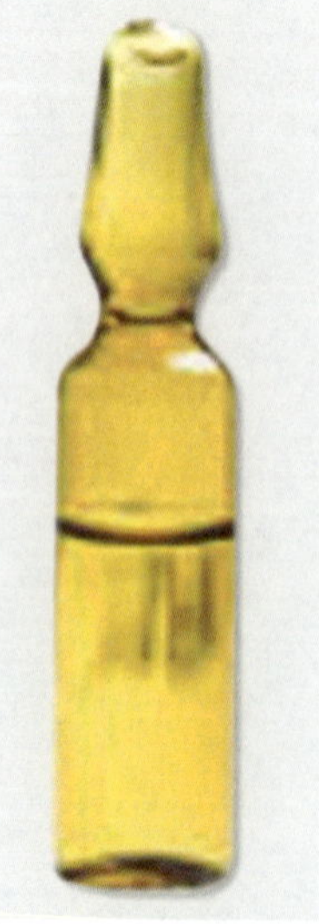

Ampoule

Multidose Vial

Vials are small glass containers containing multiple doses of a liquid medicine meant for parenteral administration. It is sealed with a rubber cap that permits needle insertion for multiple doses. Aseptic precautions must be followed every time. A new needle must be used every time. It should be discarded after 28 days of opening unless advised otherwise by the manufacturer.

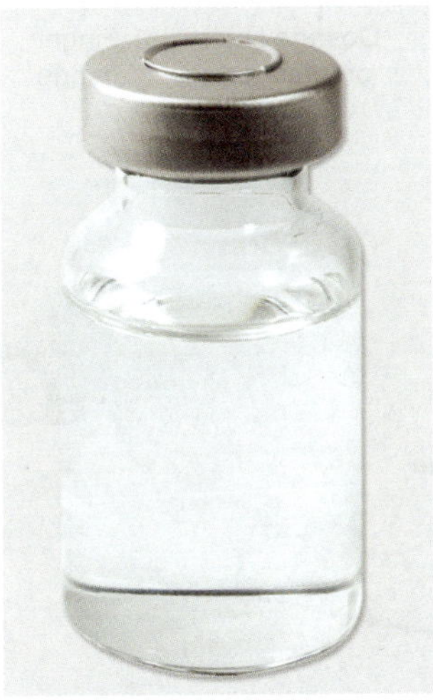

Multidose vial

Infusion Bags/Bottles

Aqueous solutions in volumes of 100–5,000 mL (large volume parenteral) are available in infusion bags or bottles for IV administration.

IV fluids are broadly classified as:

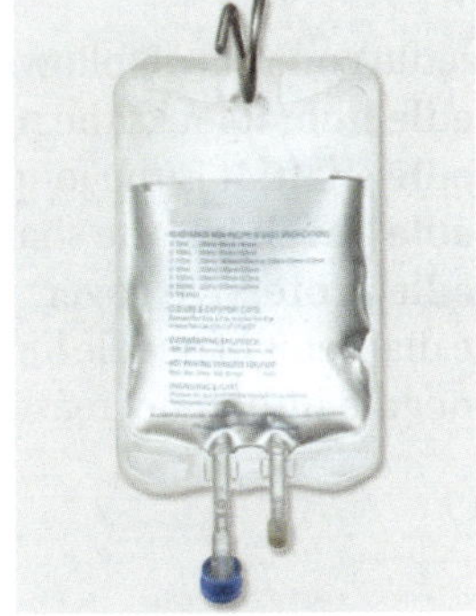

Infusion bags/bottles

Crystalloids

They consist of small dissoluble molecules that easily pass into bloodstream and tissue cells. They are generally used for rehydration and postoperative hydration.

- Normal saline (9%)—sodium chloride in water
- 5%, 10%, 20% dextrose—dextrose in water
- Ringer lactate—sodium, potassium, calcium, chloride and lactate

Colloids

They consist of large molecules that cannot easily pass through cell membrane and stay mainly in bloodstream, e.g., albumin, hespan. They are used for shock, external burns, pancreatitis, etc.

DRUG DELIVERY DEVICES FOR PARENTERAL DRUG ADMINISTRATION

Syringes and Needles

Syringes and needles are sterile devices that are used to inject medications or fluids into the body or withdraw body fluids.

Syringe

Syringe is made up of three parts:

1. **Plunger:** It is pushed and pulled inside the barrel in order to draw in or expel the fluid.
2. **Barrel:** It is the cylindrical part of the syringe that holds the fluid.
3. **Luer lock:** It is a screw-shaped structure that allows the needle to be attached on the tip of syringe and locked. Many syringes are also available without Luer lock.

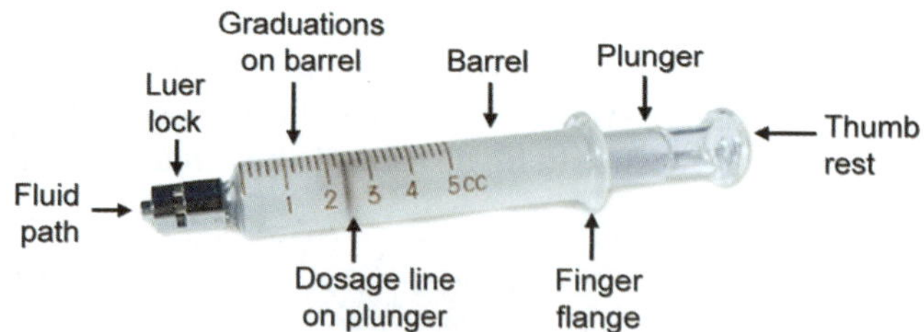

Parts of syringe

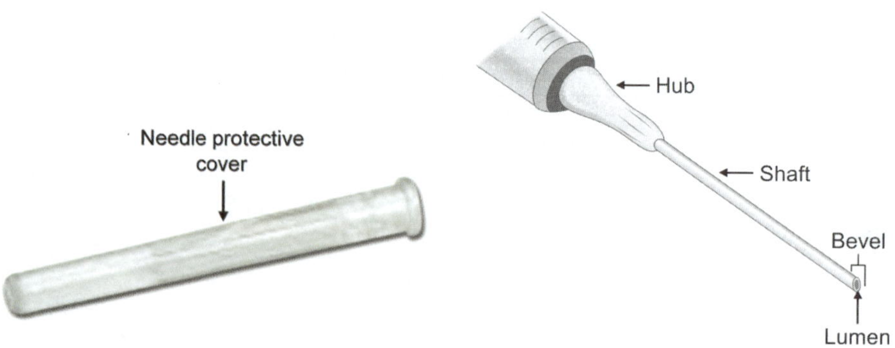

Parts of needle

Needle

The needle consists of following parts:

- **Needle hub:** It locks the needle in place while using a syringe.
- **Needle shaft:** It is the long slender stem of the needle.
- **Needle bevel:** It is the sharpened and angle shaped area at the tip that is used for puncturing tissue.
- **Needle protective cover**

The diameter of needle lumen may range from 6 gauge to 34 gauge. As the needle gauge number increases the diameter of the needle lumen decreases or narrows down.

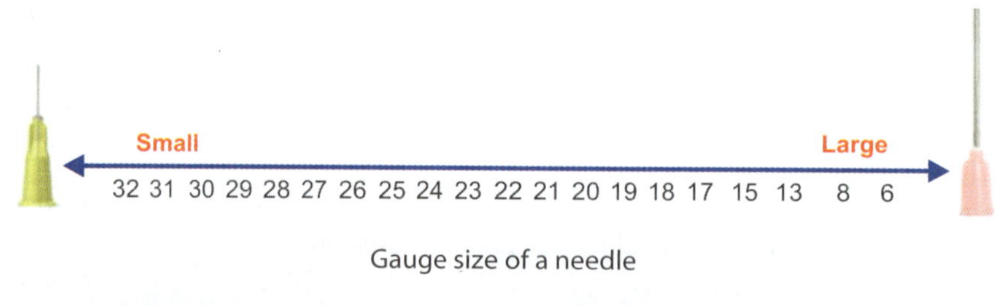

Gauge size of a needle

30 G	29 G	28 G	27 G	26 G	25 G	24 G	23 G	22 G	21 G	20 G	19 G	18 G

ISO Hub Color Code Standards for Guage Size

Needle hub color codes

Type of injection	*Size required*
Subcutaneous injection	19–27 G
Intramuscular injection	20–22 G
Intradermal injection	26–28 G
Venepuncture	21 G

Intravenous (IV) Cannula

It is a hollow tube with a sharp inner core that is inserted into a vein for administration of fluids, medicines or obtaining blood samples. IV cannulas are color coded to define the size and uses. The size of IV cannula varies from 14 to 26 Gauge.

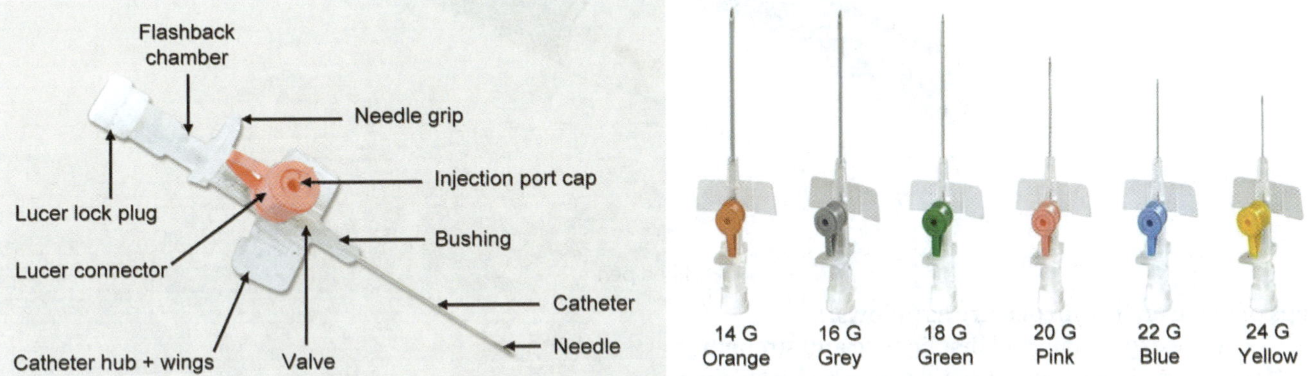

Parts of intravenous cannula

Size of IV cannula	*Recommendations*
24–26 G	Infants and neonates
22–25 G	Pediatric patients
18–20 G	Adult patients
16–18 G	Rapid transfusions in adults

Prefilled Syringe

It is a disposable syringe containing a single dose for parenteral administration. It contains a needle guard to protect from needle stick injuries. It decreases the steps of injection, decreases the risk of contamination and inaccurate dosing, e.g., enoxaparin, amiodarone.

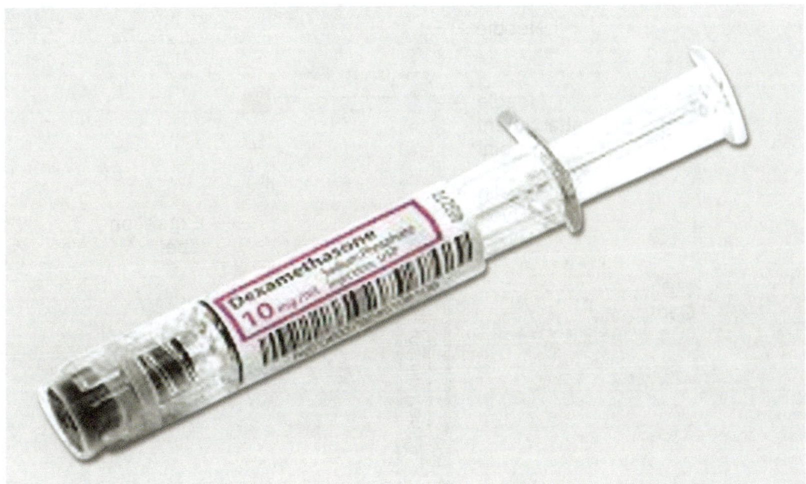

Prefilled syringe

Prefilled Pen

It is an injection device with a needle and a prefilled cartridge of medication. It can be disposable or reusable. Diabetic patients who have to take regular insulin find them less painful and more convenient.

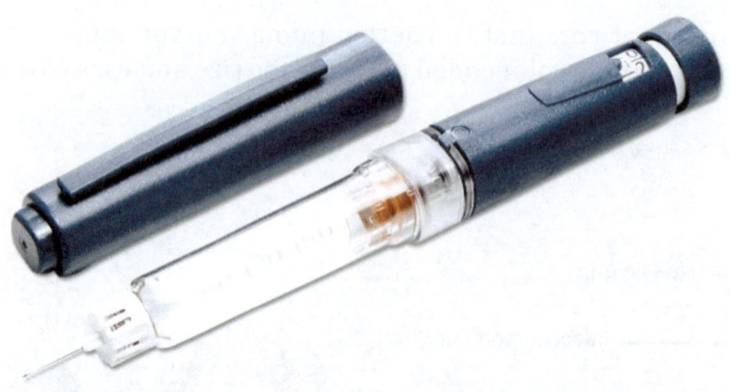

Prefilled pen

Steps of using an insulin pen are as follows:

1. Check the expiry date and insulin type and strength.
2. If necessary, insert a new cartridge into a reusable pen.
3. Mix the insulin by gently rolling the pen between the palms. Tilt the pen up and down.
4. Wash hands thoroughly.
5. Remove pen cap, and clean the top with alcohol.
6. Attach a new needle to the pen.
7. Remove the needle caps while retaining the outer cap.
8. Turn the dial to the correct dose.
9. Clean the chosen injection site with alcohol, and allow the area to dry.
10. Hold the pen to the injection site, press the injection button.
11. Wait for 10 seconds before removing the needle from the skin.
12. Press on the injection site for 5–10 seconds, but do not rub the skin.
13. Remove and safely dispose off the needle, replace the cap on the pen.

Note: Insulin pens should be kept in refrigerator. It should never be stored with a needle attached to it.

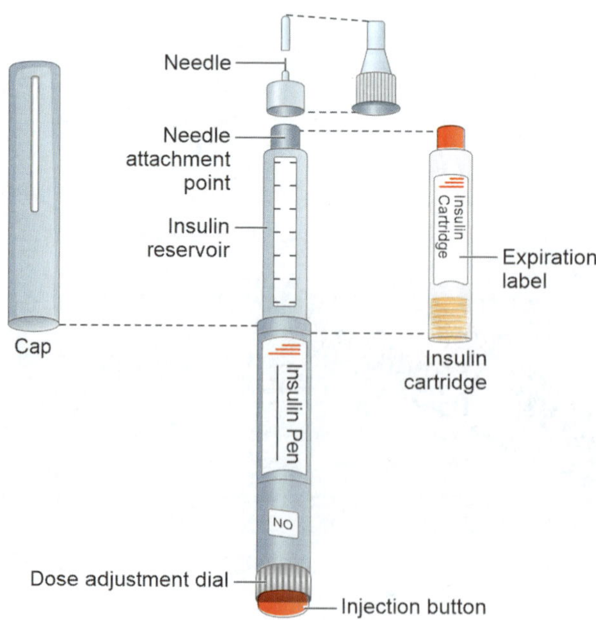

Parts of insulin pen

CONTINUOUS SUBCUTANEOUS INSULIN INFUSION PUMP

Continuous subcutaneous insulin infusion (CSII) is used in patients with type-I diabetes in order to achieve strict blood glucose control. It consists of a portable programmable electromechanical pump that infuses insulin at a basal rate continuously. Booster bolus doses are activated by the patient after food is taken. The pump contains an insulin prefilled cartridge connected to a catheter inserted subcutaneously. Newer CSII pumps also have a sensor for continuous glucose monitoring (CGM). Alarms could also be set that warn the patient about blood glucose levels too high or too low.

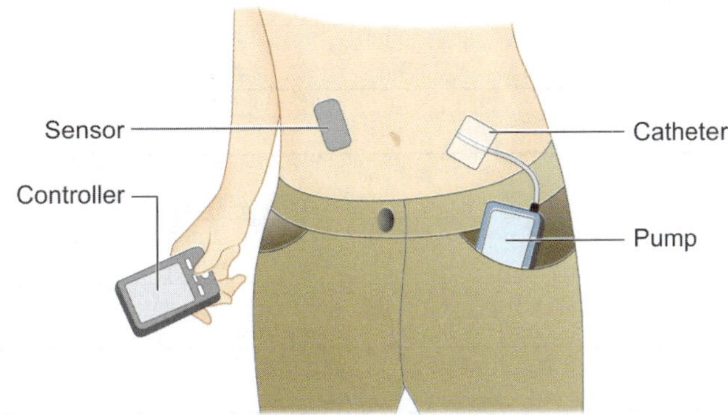

Continuous subcutaneous insulin infusion (CSII) pump

SYRINGE INFUSION PUMP

It is a small pump device that is used to accurately administer fluids with or without medicines at a controlled rate. The infusion rate and duration is programmed through a built-in software. They are used to deliver medicines like hormones, antibiotics, chemotherapeutic agents, insulin, analgesics, etc. They can also be used to deliver parenteral nutrients at controlled rate.

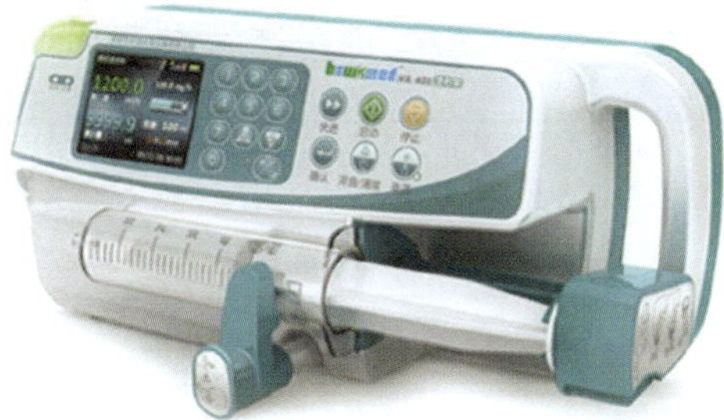

Syringe infusion pump

EXERCISES

Exercise 1: Enumerate advantages of parenteral route of drug administration.

Exercise 2: Enumerate disadvantages of parenteral route of drug administration.

Exercise 3: Enumerate difference between an ampoule and a vial.

Exercise 4: What are prefilled syringes and prefilled pen? Enumerate their uses and advantages over simple syringes.

NOTES

CHAPTER

Parenteral Drug Administration

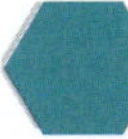

COMPETENCIES

PH1.4: Identify the common drug formulations and drug delivery systems, demonstrate their use and describe their advantages and disadvantages.
PH1.5: Describe various routes of drug administration, their advantages and disadvantages and demonstrate administration.

MANNEQUIN

A mannequin is a full-body or a part of body simulator that mimics human anatomy and physiology. It safely allows teaching of clinical skills in a professional healthcare setting.

In pharmacology, with the help of these mannequins, students can learn drug preparation and administration skills by valid and reliable methods in a student friendly environment. They help to develop both psychomotor and affective domains of learning.

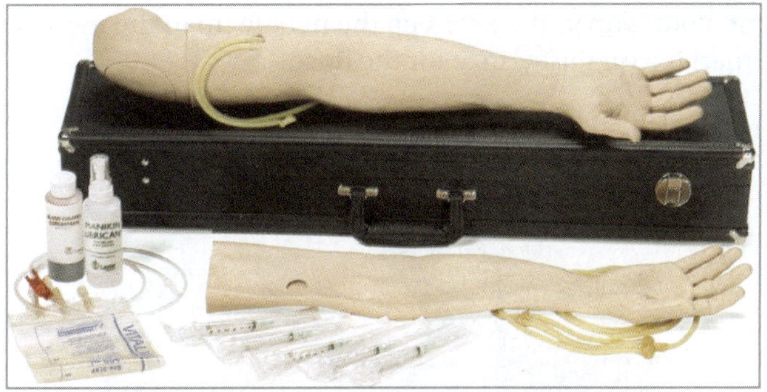

Mannequin of upper arm for parenteral drug administration

Note: In this chapter procedures of various parenteral injections have been discussed. For proper selection of syringe and needles *refer* to chapter 6.

PREPARING MEDICATIONS FROM AMPOULES OR VIALS

Medicines for parenteral administration are available in ampoules, vials or prefilled syringes.

Ampoules are glass containers for single use. Their neck has to be broken before use. A needle with filter should be preferred while aspirating fluid from ampoule to prevent glass particles drawn up in syringe. But never use a filter needle to inject.

Method of Withdrawing Fluid from an Ampoule

- Wash hands and wear gloves
- Clean the neck of ampoule with an alcohol swab
- Remove the syringe from package and attach a filter needle

- Hold the ampoule upright and tap the top to move the fluid down
- With a clean piece of gauge grasp the neck and snap it directing away
- Remove the cap of the needle and, tilting the ampoule gently, place the tip of the needle inside the ampoule, and withdraw the medication into the syringe.
- Hold the syringe straight and gently tap the side to bring any air bubbles to the top
- Gently push any air out of the syringe and recap.

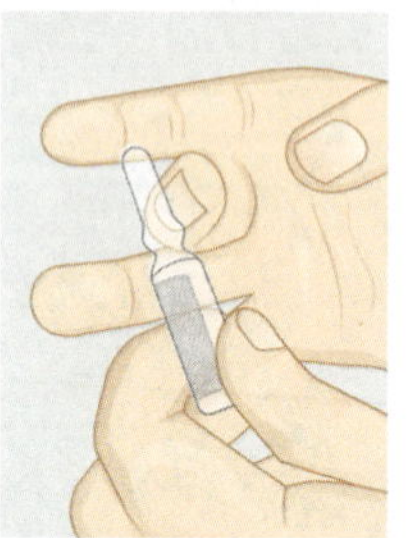

Tap to move the fluid down

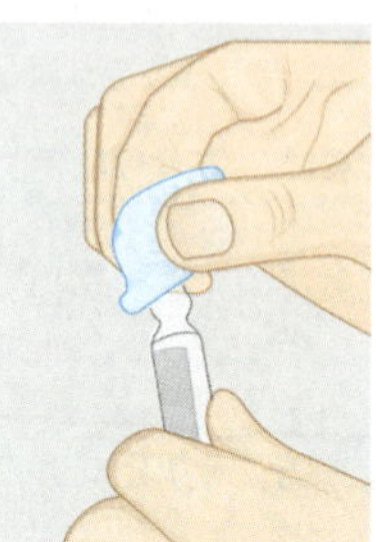

Place a gauge around the neck

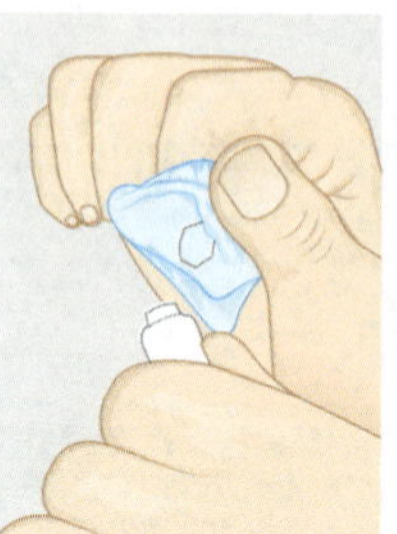

Snap the neck

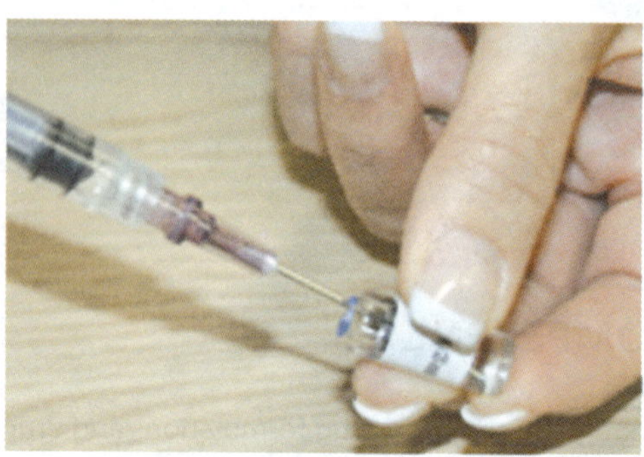

Withdrawing fluid from an ampoule

A vial is a multidose glass or plastic container with a rubber seal top.

Method of Withdrawing Fluid from a Vial

- Wash hands and wear gloves
- Hold the syringe in the hand like a pencil, with the needle pointed up.
- Pull back the plunger to the marking on the syringe for the dose, to fill the syringe with air.
- Insert the needle into the rubber top of vial. Do not touch or bend the needle.
- Push the air into the vial.
- Turn the vial upside down and hold it up in the air. Keep the needle tip in the medicine.
- Pull back the plunger to the marking on the syringe for the dose.

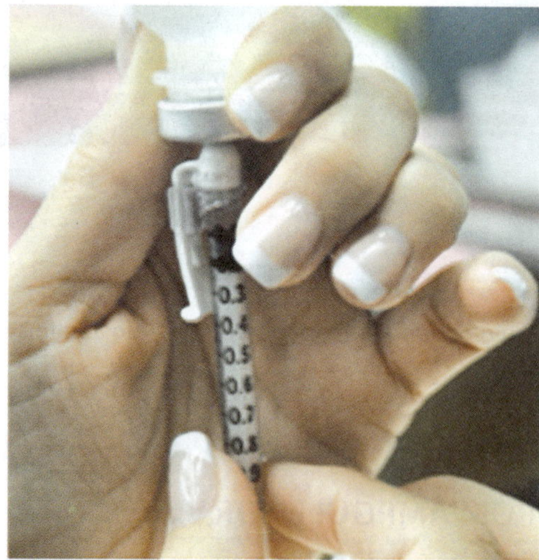

Withdrawing fluid from a vial

LEARN AND PRACTICE INTRAVENOUS INJECTION PROCEDURE

- Intravenous injection introduces a drug directly into the venous system. A drug can also be administered intravenously through an already established IV line.

- In emergency conditions, a direct IV injection can be given. Medicine given via IV route should be administered very slowly taking one minute.
- **Common sites:** On ventral aspect of elbow or forearm, median cubital, basilic or cephalic veins are used. On dorsal aspect of forearm, brachial, cephalic or metacarpal veins are used.
- **Dose:** Maximum 20 mL
- **Complications:** Extravasation, hematoma, air embolism, thrombophlebitis, intra-arterial injection (unintended)

Steps to be Followed

1. Explain the procedure to patient, confirm consent
2. Make sure you have the right amount of the right medicine in the right syringe and needle.
3. Perform hand hygiene and wear gloves
4. Prepare the patient in correct position and carefully locate the site for injection
5. Remove air from the syringe by holding the syringe in upright position and gently pressing the piston until a drop of solution comes to the tip of the needle
6. Select a suitable superficial vein.
7. Wrap a tourniquet (usually on the upper arm) to fill the peripheral veins. Visualizing a vein can be facilitated by warming the limb and massaging (tapping) the planned injection site.
8. Spread the skin taut below the planned injection site using a thumb or fingers of one hand. Alternatively ask the patient to open and close their fist several times.
9. Clean the site with an alcohol or antiseptic swab using a firm, circular motion. Start disinfecting over the planned injection site and move outwards in circular motion. Allow the site to dry completely.
10. Spread the skin taut below the planned injection site using the thumb and fingers of one hand. Insert the needle with a syringe attached into the skin at a ~30° angle, simultaneously aspirating the syringe plunger.
11. When blood is seen in the syringe, release the tourniquet and inject the drug slowly, then withdraw the needle.
12. Compress the injection site with a sterile gauze immediately after the needle is removed to stop bleeding, then protect it with a small adhesive dressing.
13. Discard the needle and syringe as per biomedical waste management rules.

LEARN AND PRACTICE INTRAMUSCULAR INJECTION PROCEDURE

- Intramuscular injection deposits medicine into the muscle fascia which has a rich blood supply.
- **Common sites**
  - *Ventrogluteal site:* Most preferred site as it is free from blood vessels and nerves, and compared to other sites muscle thickness is greatest. It is also preferable for administration of oily and irritating substances. Up to 3 mL of drug can be given.

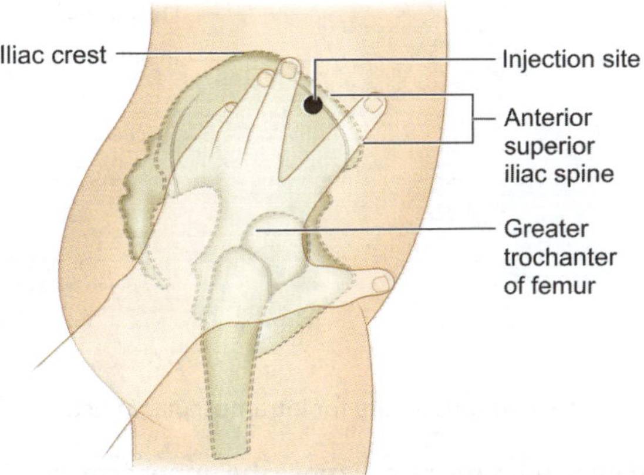

Ventrogluteal site for intramuscular injection

- How to locate ventrogluteal site: Place the patient in a supine or lateral position. The right hand is used for the left hip, and the left for the right hip. Place the heel or palm of hand on the greater trochanter, with the thumb pointed toward the belly button. Extend the index finger to the anterior superior iliac spine and spread the middle finger pointing towards the iliac crest. Insert the needle into the 'V' formed between the index and the middle fingers.

➢ *Vastus lateralis site:* It is commonly used for immunization in children. Up to 3 mL fluid can be given.

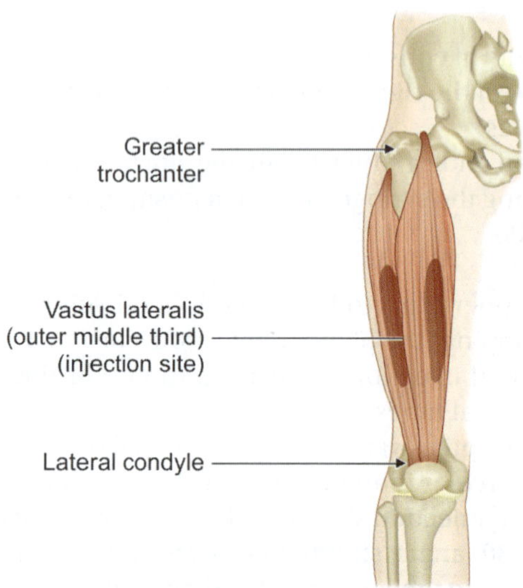

Vastus lateralis site for intramuscular injection

- How to locate: Ask the patient to lie flat with knees slightly bent, or in a sitting position. It is located on the anterior lateral aspect of the thigh and extends from one hand's breadth above the knee to one hand's breadth below the greater trochanter. The middle third of the muscle is used for injections. The width used extends from the midline of the thigh to the midline of the outer thigh.

➢ *Deltoid muscle site:* It is triangular shaped site in arm and easy to locate and injection can be given in standing, sitting or lying down position. Maximum amount that can be injected at one time is 1 mL.

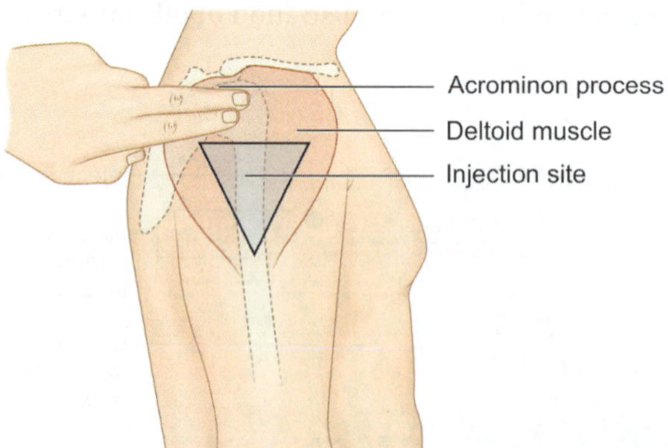

Deltoid muscle site for intramuscular injection

- How to locate: Ask the patient to relax the arm. Expose the upper arm and find the acromion process by palpating the bony prominence. The injection site is in the middle of the deltoid muscle, about 2.5–5 cm (1–2 inches) below the acromion process. Lay three fingers across the deltoid muscle and below the acromion process. The injection site is generally three finger widths below, in the middle of the muscle.

Special Considerations

- ❖ Choose a site that is free from infection, abrasions, or necrosis.
- ❖ Avoid emaciated or atrophied muscles as they absorb medications poorly.
- ❖ Rotate the site if frequent injections are given to decrease the risk of hypertrophy.
- ❖ Older adults and thin patients may only tolerate up to 2 mL in a single injection.

Complications

Muscle atrophy, injury to bone, cellulitis, sterile abscess, nerve injury, and risk of direct injection into bloodstream.

Steps to be Followed

1. Explain the procedure to patient, confirm consent
2. Make sure you have the right amount of the right medicine in the right syringe.
3. Perform hand hygiene and wear gloves
4. Prepare the patient in correct position and carefully locate the site for injection
5. Clean the skin with an alcohol or antiseptic swab. Let it dry.
6. Take the cap off the needle. Hold syringe between thumb and forefinger on dominant hand as if holding a dart.
7. Hold the skin around the injection site with the thumb and index finger of nondominant hand.
8. Inject the needle quickly into the muscle at a 90° angle, using a steady and smooth motion.
9. Use the thumb and forefinger of the nondominant hand to hold the syringe
10. Aspirate for blood and if no blood appears, inject the medication slowly and steadily.
11. Pull the needle straight out and press the site with a sterile gauge or band-aid.

Z-track Method

A zigzag path is created to prevent medication from leaking into the subcutaneous tissue. Displace skin in a Z-track manner by pulling the skin down or to one side about 2 cm with the nondominant hand and quickly insert needle at a 90° angle. Continue pulling on skin with nondominant hand, and at the same time grasp lower end of syringe barrel with fingers of nondominant hand to stabilize it. Move dominant hand to end of plunger. If required, aspirate for blood and if no blood appears, inject the medication slowly. Leave the needle in place for 10 seconds. Remove the needle using a smooth, steady motion, and then release the skin.

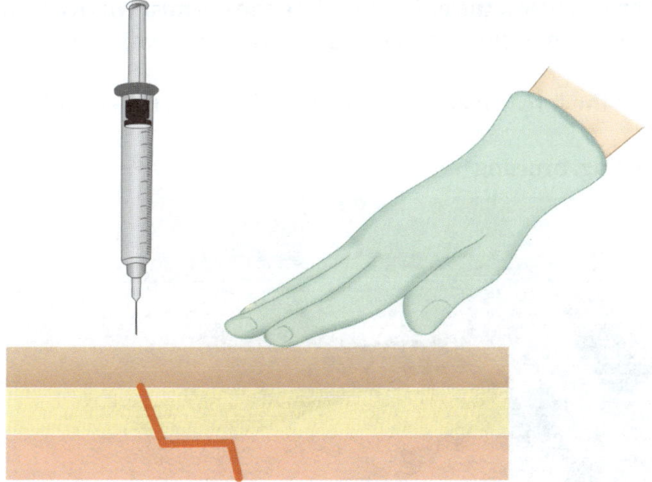

Z-track method of intramuscular injection

LEARN AND PRACTICE SUBCUTANEOUS INJECTION PROCEDURE

- ❖ Subcutaneous (SC) injections are administered just below the epidermis and dermis, into the adipose tissue layer.
- ❖ This route is commonly used to administer insulin, heparin, opioids and adrenaline.

- Physical exercise or hot or cold compress application modifies the rate of drug absorption by modifying the local blood flow.
- It is advisable to rotate the site to prevent lipohypertrophy or lipoatrophy.
- **Common sites:** Outer aspect of the upper arm, the abdomen within one inch of the umbilicus, anterior aspects of the thighs, upper back, and upper ventral gluteal area. The site should be free from any skin lesion and bony prominences.
- **Dose:** Less than 1 mL
- **Complications:** Infection, abscess, swelling, redness, bruising, intravenous injection

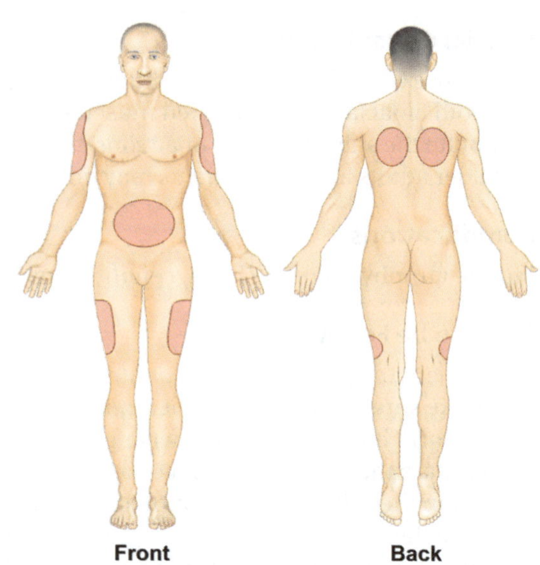

Common sites for subcutaneous injection

Steps for Subcutaneous Injection

1. Explain the procedure to the patient, confirm consent.
2. Make sure you have the right amount of the right medicine in the right syringe.
3. Perform hand hygiene and wear gloves.
4. Clean the site with an alcohol or antiseptic swab using a firm, circular motion. Allow the site to dry.
5. Remove needle from cap by pulling it off in a straight motion.
6. Pinch the skin surrounding the injection site, or spread the skin taut at the site between your thumb and index finger.
7. Hold the syringe in the dominant hand between the thumb and forefinger and insert the needle quickly at a 45–90° angle. Inserting quickly causes less pain to the patient.
8. After the needle is in place, release the tissue and move the nondominant hand to steady the needle. With the dominant hand, inject the medication at a rate of 10 seconds per mL without moving the syringe.
9. Withdraw the needle quickly at the same angle while supporting the surrounding tissue with the nondominant hand.
10. Apply gentle pressure at the site with a sterile gauge. Do not massage the site.

LEARN AND PRACTICE INTRADERMAL INJECTION PROCEDURE

- Intradermal injections are given just below the epidermis, into the dermis. This route is commonly used for sensitivity test. Injection site should be free from lesions, rashes, moles, or scars, which may alter the visual inspection of the test results.
- **Common sites:** Inner surface of the forearm and the upper back, under the scapula
- **Dose:** 0.01–0.1 mL (<0.5 mL)
- **Complications:** Infection, swelling, bruising

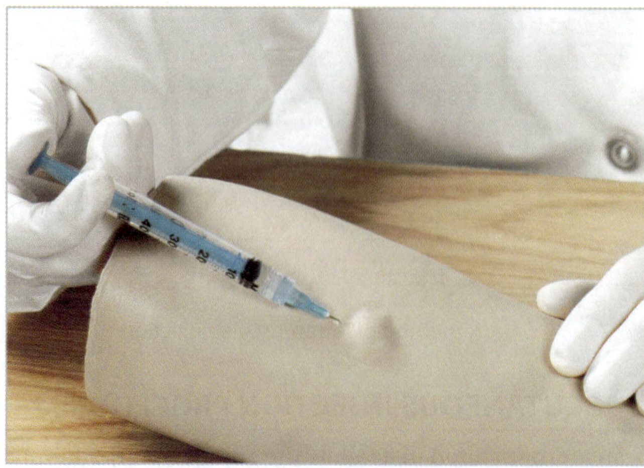

Intradermal injection on a mannequin

Steps to be Followed

1. Explain the procedure to the patient, confirm consent.
2. Make sure you have the right amount of the right medicine in the right syringe.
3. Perform hand hygiene and wear gloves.
4. Clean the site with an alcohol or antiseptic swab using a firm, circular motion. Allow the site to dry.
5. Remove needle from cap by pulling it off in a straight motion.
6. Spread the skin taut over the injection site with the non-dominant hand.
7. Hold syringe at a 5–15° angle from the site. Place the needle almost flat against the patient's skin, bevel side up, and insert needle into the skin. Insert the needle only about 1/4 inch, with the entire bevel under the skin.
8. Slowly inject the solution. This will raise a small bleb on the site.
9. Withdraw the needle at the same angle as insertion.
10. Do not clean or massage area after injection.

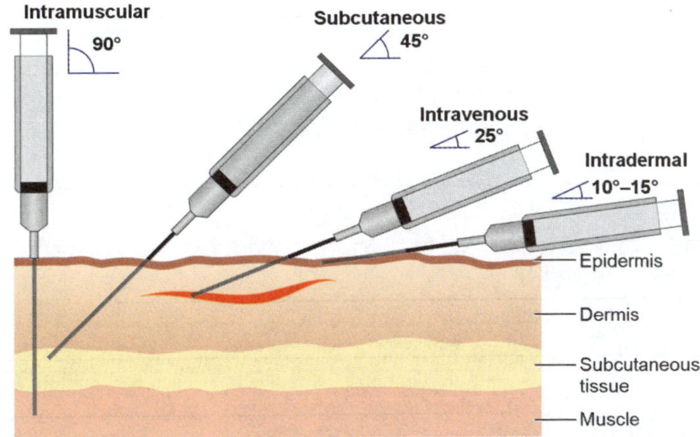

Angles of insertion for different parenteral injections

EXERCISES

Exercise 1: Administer intravenous injection in a mannequin following all steps, and enumerate the steps below.

Exercise 2: Administer intramuscular injection in a mannequin following all the steps, and enumerate the steps below.

Exercise 3: Administer subcutaneous injection in a mannequin following all the steps, and enumerate the steps below.

Exercise 4: Administer intradermal injection in a mannequin following all the steps, and enumerate the steps below.

**Above exercises should be performed in a simulated environment using psychomotor and affective skills.

Reference: Doyle GR, McCutcheon JA. Clinical Procedures for Safer Patient Care. Victoria, BC: BCcampus, 2015. Retrieved from https://opentextbc.ca/clinicalskills/

NOTES

CHAPTER

8

Setting an Intravenous Drip

COMPETENCIES

PH1.4: Identify the common drug formulations and drug delivery systems, demonstrate their use and describe their advantages and disadvantages.
PH1.5: Describe various routes of drug administration, their advantages and disadvantages and demonstrate administration.

INTRAVENOUS INFUSION

It is a method of administering fluids and medicines into the bloodstream through a vein.

INTRAVENOUS INFUSION EQUIPMENT

Intravenous (IV) fluids and medications are administered to patients by using an IV infusion set which consists of flexible plastic tubing. This set connects the bag of solution to the intravenous access site of the patient.

Primary IV Infusion Set

This set is used to administer intermittent or continuous IV fluids or medications to the patient. Following are the parts of primary IV set:

- **Spike:** This end of tube is entered into the fluid bag. It should be kept sterile. It is also known as plunger.
- **Plastic tubing:** Flexible plastic tube for passage of fluid.
- **Drip chamber:** It is helpful in calculating the drip rate, i.e., drops/minute. It also helps to prevent air bubbles in tubing to move further. It should be kept half filled with solution.
- **Access port:** This is also known as 'Y' port. This is for administration of additional medication. In some sets a latex tube is connected instead of 'Y' port.
- **Roller clamp/regulator:** This helps in controlling the drip rate.
- **Needle adapter:** This end is connected to the needle that enters in the patient's vein.

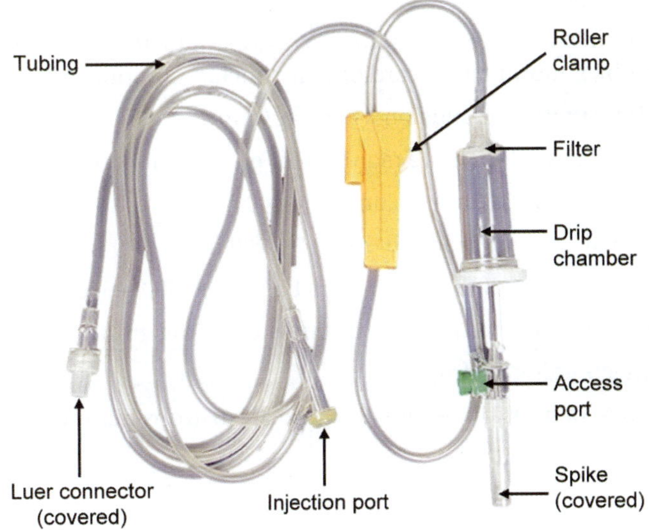

Components of intravenous infusion set

Secondary IV Infusion Set

This is used to administer a second medication, e.g., an antibiotic, while primary medication is also being given IV. Its tubing is shorter in length and is attached to the primary line with the access port.

Procedure for Setting an IV Drip

- Follow aseptic precautions.
- Explain the procedure to patients, and take consent.
- Check the fluid bag for any cloudiness or particulate matter.
- Remove the outer packing of the fluid bag.
- Open the IV set and with the help of roller clamp close the flow control.
- Remove the cover on the entry port on the fluid bag by twisting it.
- Insert the spike into entry port in fluid bag without touching the spike with hand. Now hang the fluid bag on the drip stand with the help of a hook.
- Half fill the drip chamber by squeezing the fluid bag.
- Release the roller clamp to allow the fluid to pass through the set.
- Ensure that there are no bubbles in the tubing. Again, bring the roller clamp to the lower end.
- Perform venepuncture following all aseptic precautions and then connect the needle adapter to the venous cannula. Take care that there are no air bubbles.
- Open the roller clamp and adjust the flow rate as per requirement.

Complications of IV Infusion

- **Extravasation of IV fluid in the surrounding tissue:** This can cause tissue injury depending on the drug and length of exposure.
- **Necrosis:** In rare cases it may cause tissue necrosis on leakage into surrounding tissue, e.g., noradrenaline drip.
- **Thrombophlebitis:** Inflammation of superficial vein
- **Infection and sepsis:** It may occur if proper aseptic precautions are not followed.

Calculation of Drip Rate

This includes calculation of the number of drops allowed to enter the drip chamber per minute. It is set manually and it determines the rate of fluid entering into patient's body.

- Calculate the total dose required according to the body weight of the patient
- Calculate drug concentration in IV fluid to be administered
- Now calculate drops per minute to be administered to the patient, keeping in mind that 1 mL contains 20 drops or 60 microdrops.

Example: Prepare an IV infusion of dopamine to deliver 2 µg/kg/minute for a 50-year-old patient Suresh Kumar of 60 kg weight, suffering from cardiogenic shock. 1 ampoule of 5 mL contains 40 mg/mL of dopamine.

Solution: Rate of infusion = 2 µg/kg/min

Total dose of dopamine required for given patient of 60 kg weight = 60 × 2 = 120 µg/min

1 ampoule of dopamine containing 40 mg/mL is added in 500 mL infusion bag of dextrose

So, total dopamine added = 40 × 5 = 200 mg in 500 mL of dextrose = 200,000 µg in 500 mL

Concentration of drug in IV fluid bag = 2,00,000 ÷ 500 = 400 µg/mL

Rate of infusion required to administer 120 µg/min = 120 ÷ 400 = 0.3 mL/min

1 mL contains 20 drops

So, rate of infusion required = 0.3 × 20 = 6 drops per minute

EXERCISES

Exercise 1: Prepare an IV infusion of dopamine to deliver 5 µg/kg/minute for a 52-year-old patient Kamlesh Singh of 60 kg body weight, suffering from cardiogenic shock. 1 ampoule of 5 mL contains 40 mg/mL of dopamine.

Exercise 2: Calculate the IV infusion rate (drops per minute) for noradrenaline drip, to deliver 0.1 µg/kg/minute to a 40-year-old female patient weighing 60 kg, suffering from septic shock.

1 ampoule of noradrenaline contains 2 mg base and 2 ampoules were added in 500 mL of 5% dextrose.

NOTES

NOTES

CHAPTER

9

Pharmacovigilance and Adverse Drug Reaction Monitoring

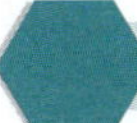

COMPETENCIES

PH1.11: Define adverse drug reactions (ADRs) and their types. Identify the ADRs in the given case scenario and assess causality.
PH1.12: Define pharmacovigilance, its principles and demonstrate ADR reporting.

PHARMACOVIGILANCE

WHO defines pharmacovigilance as the science and activities related to the detection, assessment, understanding and prevention of adverse effects or any other medicine or vaccine-related problems.

What is the need of Pharmacovigilance?

All medicines and vaccines are rigorously tested in clinical trials before they are allowed to be used in human beings. These clinical trials are done on selected number of patients (few hundred), in controlled environment and for a limited period of time. There is still a risk of unknown adverse effect from drug when it is given to a heterogeneous population for a long period of time and with concurrent illnesses.

Thus, there is a need to keep a continuous vigilance on adverse drug effects.

Pharmacovigilance Programme of India (PvPI)

- National program run by Central Drug Standard Control Organization (CDSCO), under the aegis of Ministry of Health and Family Welfare, Government of India. This program was launched in 2010.
- **National Coordination Centre (NCC):** Indian Pharmacopoeia Commission (IPC), Ghaziabad, Uttar Pradesh.
- NCC also works as WHO Collaborating Centre for Pharmacovigilance in Public Health Program and Regulatory Services.

Mission

To safeguard the health of the population of India by ensuring safe use of medicines.

Purpose

To collect and analyze data and use the inferences to recommend informed regulatory interventions, and to communicate risks to healthcare professionals and public.

Materiovigilance Programme of India (MvPI)

This program has been developed for monitoring of adverse events related to medical devices. This program is also coordinated by IPC, Ghaziabad.

Adverse Drug Event

Any adverse event that could be related to medicine(s) taken by the patient is considered adverse drug event. Causality assessment helps in determining the chances of that event occurring as a result of medicine or disease or some other condition.

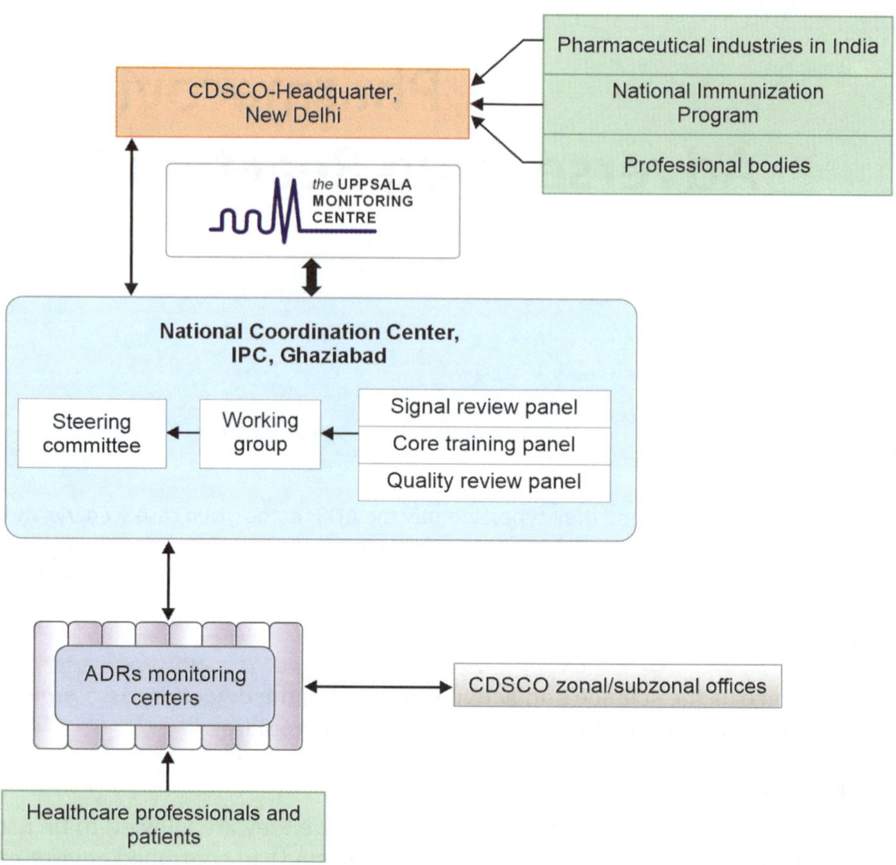

(ADRs: adverse drug reactions; CDSCO: Central Drugs Standard Control Organization; IPC: Indian Pharmacopoeia Commission)

Source: https://ipc.gov.in/PvPI/about.html

Adverse Drug Reaction

WHO has defined ADR as a response that is noxious and unintended, and that occurs at doses normally used in humans for the prophylaxis, diagnosis, or therapy of disease, or for the modification of physiological function. Recent modifications also allow inclusion of reactions occurring due to error, misuse, abuse, off-label use and use of unlicensed medicines.

ADRs are broadly classified as follows:

- **Type A reactions**: They are also known as augmented or predictable reactions. They are related to the pharmacological properties of the drug and thus dose related and predictable. Type A reactions include side effects and toxic effects.
- **Type B reactions**: They are also known as bizarre or unpredictable reactions. These reactions cannot be defined by drug's pharmacological properties and are thus unpredictable and often nondose related. Type B reactions include allergic and idiosyncratic reactions.
- **Type C reactions**: They are also known as 'continuing reactions'. These reactions occur due to continuous or persistent use of a drug for a long time.
- **Type D reactions**: They are also known as 'delayed reactions'. These reactions become apparent sometime after the use of drug, e.g., teratogenic effects.
- **Type E reactions**: They are also known as 'end of use' reactions. These include withdrawal reactions.

Dechallenge

This refers to stopping of the drug after appearance of an adverse drug event. If the adverse event subsides after stopping the drug, it is termed as dechallenge is positive. If the adverse event does not subside even after stopping the drug, it is termed as negative dechallenge.

Rechallenge

This refers to restarting the drug after it has been stopped due to an adverse drug event. If the same adverse reaction reappears, it is termed as positive rechallenge. If the adverse reaction does not reappear after restarting the drug, it is termed as negative rechallenge.

Diagnosis of ADRs

A drug related adverse event may present itself in varied forms including physical sign and symptoms, biochemical or hematological derangements. A comprehensive medication history is most important to identify adverse drug reactions. Clinician should enquire about any prior exposure with the suspected drug, time relation of ADR with suspected drug, over-the-counter (OTC) medicine and complementary and alternative medicine (CAM). In some cases, laboratory investigations can help in diagnosis of ADR, e.g., rifampicin-induced hepatitis.

Management of ADRs

The most common approach is alteration in dosage regimen or withdrawal of offending drug (s). The management ADRs also depends on specific drug responsible, e.g., naloxone is given for opioid-induced toxicity. Benefit risk assessment is also important while managing ADRs. Sometimes minor ADRs of life-saving drugs are managed with symptomatic treatment, e.g., antiemetics for cancer chemotherapy induced nausea and vomiting.

Prevention of ADRs

Some ADRs are unpredictable, e.g., anaphylactic reaction, but many can be prevented. Some general measures that could be adopted in order to prevent ADRs are as follows:

- Medication history—a proper medication history from every patient helps in identifying previous ADRs and precludes re-exposure with those drugs
- Avoid polypharmacy
- Treatment plan should consider possible adverse effects, e.g., pyridoxine should be coprescribed with isoniazid to prevent neurotoxicity
- Cautious prescribing and monitoring in patient with hepatic or renal insufficiency
- Therapeutic drug monitoring
- Pharmacogenomic analysis could help in identifying individuals that are at high risk of toxicity from certain drugs

Causality Assessment/Analysis

It is a method of analysis of ADEs, to know the strength of relationship between adverse event and drug exposure. It is usually done by a committee of experts in the institute where Suspected Adverse Drug Reaction Reporting Forms (SADRRF) are collected in ADR monitoring center. For such analysis specific causality assessment tools are used.

Common causality assessment tools available for causality assessment:

- **World Health Organization:** Uppsala Monitoring Center (WHO-UMC) scale
- Naranjo ADR probability scale
- Swedish method
- Bayesian Adverse Reaction Diagnostic Instrument (BARDI)

WHO-UMC Scale

This scale is used for causality assessment under PvPI. It categorizes an ADR into the following categories:

Causality terms	*Assessment criteria*
Certain	• Event or laboratory test abnormality, with plausible time relationship to drug intake • Cannot be explained by disease or other drugs • Response to withdrawal plausible (pharmacologically, pathologically) • Event definitive pharmacologically or phenomenologically (i.e., an objective and specific medical disorder or a recognized pharmacological phenomenon) • Rechallenge satisfactory, if necessary

Contd....

Contd....

Causality terms	*Assessment criteria*
Probable/likely	• Event or laboratory test abnormality, with reasonable time relationship to drug intake • Unlikely to be attributed to disease or other drugs • Response to withdrawal clinically reasonable • Rechallenge not required
Possible	• Event or laboratory test abnormality, with reasonable time relationship to drug intake • Could also be explained by disease or other drugs • Information on drug withdrawal may be lacking or unclear
Unlikely	• Event or laboratory test abnormality, with a time to drug intake that makes a relationship improbable (but not impossible) • Disease or other drugs provide plausible explanations
Conditional/unclassified	• Event or laboratory test abnormality • More data for proper assessment needed • Additional data under examination
Unassessable/unclassifiable	• Report suggesting an adverse reaction • Cannot be judged because information is insufficient or contradictory • Data cannot be supplemented or verified

Who should report ADR?

- All healthcare professionals, e.g., doctors, nurses, pharmacists, etc.
- Pharmaceutical manufacturers
- Patients, their relatives/caregivers

What to report?

All suspected adverse drug reactions, known or unknown, serious or non-serious, should be reported. A serious adverse event must be reported within twenty four hours of occurrence.

Where to report?

- A duly filled SADRRF can be submitted to the nearest ADR monitoring center (AMC) or it can be directly sent to NCC via email at pvpi@ipcindia.net or pvpi.ipcindia@gmail.com.
- ADRs can be reported to a toll-free helpline number 1800 180 3024

What happens to the submitted SADRRFs?

SADRRFs are kept in strict confidence. Causality assessment is done at AMCs by using WHO-UMC scale. The analyzed forms are forwarded to the NCC through 'Vigiflow Software'. Data is analyzed at NCC and sent to WHO Uppsala Monitoring Center in Sweden. The information generated on the basis of these SADRRFs helps in continuous assessment of the benefit-risk ratio of medicines. The information is submitted to the Steering committee of PvPI constituted by the Ministry of Health and Family Welfare. The Committee reviews the data and suggests any intervention required.

EXERCISES

Exercise 1: A 42-year-old female Shanta Devi was diagnosed with enteric fever on 2nd Jan 2022. She was prescribed Injection ceftriaxone 2 g intravenously twice a day along with tablet paracetamol 500 mg three times a day. 1st dose of ceftriaxone was given on 2nd Jan at 6:00 PM, followed which she developed maculopapular rash all over the body. She was immediately given 25 mg of tablet pheniramine. Next dose of ceftriaxone was not given; instead she was prescribed tablet levofloxacin 500 mg twice a day. The reaction almost disappeared in one hour.

Report the adverse event in the given SADRRF

Version 1.4

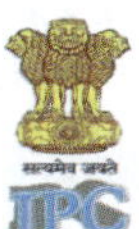

SUSPECTED ADVERSE DRUG REACTION REPORTING FORM

For **VOLUNTARY** reporting of ADRs by Healthcare Professionals

INDIAN PHARMACOPOEIA COMMISSION (National Coordination Centre-Pharmacovigilance Programme of India)

Ministry of Health & Family Welfare, Government of India, Sector-23, Raj Nagar, Ghaziabad-201002

PvPI Helpline (Toll Free) :1800-180-3024 (9:00 AM to 5:30 PM, Monday-Friday)

Initial Case ❑	Follow-up Case ❑

FOR AMC / NCC USE ONLY

Reg. No. / IPD No. / OPD No. / CR No. :

AMC Report No. :

Worldwide Unique No. :

A. PATIENT INFORMATION *

1. Patient Initials:	**2.** Age or date of birth:
3. Gender: M ❑ F ❑ Other ❑	**4.**Weight (in Kg.)

B. SUSPECTED ADVERSE REACTION *

5. Event / Reaction start date (dd/mm/yyyy)	
6. Event / Reaction stop date (dd/mm/yyyy)	

7. Describe Event/Reaction management with details , if any

12. Relevant investigations with dates :

13. Relevant medical / medication history (e.g. allergies, pregnancy, addiction, hepatic, renal dysfunction etc.)

14. Seriousness of the reaction : No❑ if Yes ❑ (*please tick anyone*)

❑Death (dd/mm/yyyy) ❑Congenital-anomaly
❑Life threatening ❑Disability
❑Hospitalization-Initial/Prolonged ❑Other Medically important

15. Outcome:

❑Recovered ❑Recovering ❑Not Recovered
❑Fatal ❑Recovered with sequelae ❑Unknown

C. SUSPECTED MEDICATION(S) *

S. No.	8. Name (Brand/ Generic)	Manufacturer (if known)	Batch No. / Lot No.	Expiry Date (if known)	Dose	Route	Frequency	Therapy Dates: Date Started	Therapy Dates: Date Stopped	Indication	Causality Assessment
i											
ii											
iii											
iv#											

9. Action taken after reaction (*please tick*)

S. No. as per C	Drug withdrawn	Dose increased	Dose reduced	Dose not changed	Not applicable	Unknown
i						
ii						
iii						
iv						

10. Reaction reappeared after reintroduction of suspected medication (*please tick*)

Yes	No	Effect unknown	Dose (if re-introduced)

11. Concomitant medical product including self-medication and herbal remedies with therapy dates (Exclude those used to treat reaction)

S. No.	Name (Brand / Generic)	Dose	Route	Frequency (OD, BD, etc.)	Therapy Dates: Date Started	Therapy Dates: Date Stopped	Indication
i							
ii							
iii#							

Additional Information :

D. REPORTER DETAILS *

16. Name & Address : ____

____

Pin : __________ Email : ____________________________________

Contact No- : ______________________________

Occupation : ____________________Signature : __________________

17. Date of this report (dd/mm/yyyy) :

Signature and Name of Receiving Personnel :

Confidentiality : The patient's identity is held in strict confidence and protected to the fullest extent. Submission of a report does not constitute an admission that medical personnel or manufacturer or the product caused or contributed to the reaction. Submission of an ADR report does not have any legal implication on the reporter.

Use separate page for more information

* Mandatory Fields for suspected ADR Reporting Form

Exercise 2: A 61-year-old patient Ram Lal presented in Medicine OPD on 15th August 2020 with complaints of muscle pain and tenderness in both legs for last fifteen days. He was a known case of ischemic heart disease and was taking tablet atorvastatin 20 mg once daily and tablet aspirin 150 mg once daily, since last six months. His CPK values were 200 µg/mL. Physical examination and rest of the investigations were normal.

Tablet atorvastatin was immediately stopped. He was advised to maintain good hydration and tablet Ibuprofen 400 mg was given on 'as and when' required basis for pain.

On follow up visit after five days, patient was much better with decreased intensity of muscle pain and CPK levels were within normal limits.

Report the adverse event in the given SADRRF

Version 1.4

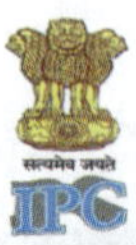

SUSPECTED ADVERSE DRUG REACTION REPORTING FORM

For **VOLUNTARY** reporting of ADRs by Healthcare Professionals

INDIAN PHARMACOPOEIA COMMISSION (National Coordination Centre-Pharmacovigilance Programme of India)

Ministry of Health & Family Welfare, Government of India, Sector-23, Raj Nagar, Ghaziabad-201002

PvPI Helpline (Toll Free) :1800-180-3024 (9:00 AM to 5:30 PM, Monday-Friday)

Initial Case ❑ | Follow-up Case ❑

FOR AMC / NCC USE ONLY

Reg. No. / IPD No. / OPD No. / CR No. :

AMC Report No. :

Worldwide Unique No. :

A. PATIENT INFORMATION *

1. Patient Initials:

2. Age or date of birth:

3. Gender: M ❑ F ❑ Other ❑

4. Weight (in Kg.)

B. SUSPECTED ADVERSE REACTION *

5. Event / Reaction start date (dd/mm/yyyy)

6. Event / Reaction stop date (dd/mm/yyyy)

7. Describe Event/Reaction management with details , if any

12. Relevant investigations with dates :

13. Relevant medical / medication history (e.g. allergies, pregnancy, addiction, hepatic, renal dysfunction etc.)

14. Seriousness of the reaction : No❑ if Yes ❑ (*please tick anyone*)

❑Death (dd/mm/yyyy) ❑Congenital-anomaly
❑Life threatening ❑Disability
❑Hospitalization-Initial/Prolonged ❑Other Medically important

15. Outcome:

❑Recovered ❑Recovering ❑Not Recovered
❑Fatal ❑Recovered with sequelae ❑Unknown

C. SUSPECTED MEDICATION(S) *

S. No.	8. Name (Brand/ Generic)	Manufacturer (if known)	Batch No. / Lot No.	Expiry Date (if known)	Dose	Route	Frequency	Therapy Dates: Date Started	Therapy Dates: Date Stopped	Indication	Causality Assessment
i											
ii											
iii											
iv#											

9. Action taken after reaction (*please tick*)

10. Reaction reappeared after reintroduction of suspected medication (*please tick*)

S. No. as per C	Drug withdrawn	Dose increased	Dose reduced	Dose not changed	Not applicable	Unknown	Yes	No	Effect unknown	Dose (if re-introduced)
i										
ii										
iii										
iv										

11. Concomitant medical product including self-medication and herbal remedies with therapy dates (Exclude those used to treat reaction)

S. No.	Name (Brand / Generic)	Dose	Route	Frequency (OD, BD, etc.)	Therapy Dates: Date Started	Therapy Dates: Date Stopped	Indication
i							
ii							
iii#							

Additional Information :

D. REPORTER DETAILS *

16. Name & Address : ____________________

Pin : __________ Email : ____________________

Contact No- : ____________________

Occupation : ____________________ Signature : ____________________

17. Date of this report (dd/mm/yyyy) :

Signature and Name of Receiving Personnel :

Confidentiality : The patient's identity is held in strict confidence and protected to the fullest extent. Submission of a report does not constitute an admission that medical personnel or manufacturer or the product caused or contributed to the reaction. Submission of an ADR report does not have any legal implication on the reporter.

Use separate page for more information

* Mandatory Fields for suspected ADR Reporting Form

Exercise 3: A 16-year-old female Sarita Yadav presented in medicine OPD on 12th January 2022 with complaint of watery diarrhea since previous night. She was also suffering from cold, cough, fever and throat pain for which she was prescribed capsule amoxicillin 500 mg three times a day and tablet paracetamol 500 mg three times a day on 11th January.

Amoxicillin was stopped and she was prescribed Tablet Azithromycin 500 mg once a day for three days. She was also given ORS powder for rehydration.

Report the adverse event in the given SADRRF.

Version 1.4

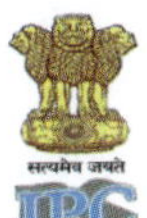

SUSPECTED ADVERSE DRUG REACTION REPORTING FORM

For **VOLUNTARY** reporting of ADRs by Healthcare Professionals

INDIAN PHARMACOPOEIA COMMISSION (National Coordination Centre-Pharmacovigilance Programme of India)

Ministry of Health & Family Welfare, Government of India, Sector-23, Raj Nagar, Ghaziabad-201002

PvPI Helpline (Toll Free) :1800-180-3024 (9:00 AM to 5:30 PM, Monday-Friday)

Initial Case ❑ | Follow-up Case ❑

FOR AMC / NCC USE ONLY

Reg. No. / IPD No. / OPD No. / CR No. :

AMC Report No. :

Worldwide Unique No. :

A. PATIENT INFORMATION *

1. Patient Initials:

2. Age or date of birth:

3. Gender: M ❑ F ❑ Other ❑

4. Weight (in Kg.)

B. SUSPECTED ADVERSE REACTION *

5. Event / Reaction start date (dd/mm/yyyy)

6. Event / Reaction stop date (dd/mm/yyyy)

7. Describe Event/Reaction management with details , if any

12. Relevant investigations with dates :

13. Relevant medical / medication history (e.g. allergies, pregnancy, addiction, hepatic, renal dysfunction etc.)

14. Seriousness of the reaction : No❑ if Yes ❑ (*please tick anyone*)

❑Death (dd/mm/yyyy) ❑Congenital-anomaly
❑Life threatening ❑Disability
❑Hospitalization-Initial/Prolonged ❑Other Medically important

15. Outcome:

❑Recovered ❑Recovering ❑Not Recovered
❑Fatal ❑Recovered with sequelae ❑Unknown

C. SUSPECTED MEDICATION(S) *

S. No.	8. Name (Brand/ Generic)	Manufacturer (if known)	Batch No. / Lot No.	Expiry Date (if known)	Dose	Route	Frequency	Therapy Dates: Date Started	Therapy Dates: Date Stopped	Indication	Causality Assessment
i											
ii											
iii											
iv#											

9. Action taken after reaction (*please tick*)

10. Reaction reappeared after reintroduction of suspected medication (*please tick*)

S. No. as per C	Drug withdrawn	Dose increased	Dose reduced	Dose not changed	Not applicable	Unknown	Yes	No	Effect unknown	Dose (if re-introduced)
i										
ii										
iii										
iv										

11. Concomitant medical product including self-medication and herbal remedies with therapy dates (Exclude those used to treat reaction)

S. No.	Name (Brand / Generic)	Dose	Route	Frequency (OD, BD, etc.)	Therapy Dates: Date Started	Therapy Dates: Date Stopped	Indication
i							
ii							
iii#							

Additional Information :

D. REPORTER DETAILS *

16. Name & Address : ______

Pin : ______ Email : ______

Contact No- : ______

Occupation : ______ Signature : ______

17. Date of this report (dd/mm/yyyy) :

Signature and Name of Receiving Personnel :

Confidentiality : The patient's identity is held in strict confidence and protected to the fullest extent. Submission of a report does not constitute an admission that medical personnel or manufacturer or the product caused or contributed to the reaction. Submission of an ADR report does not have any legal implication on the reporter.

Use separate page for more information

* Mandatory Fields for suspected ADR Reporting Form

Exercise 4: A 33-year-old male Prakash Singh presented to the skin OPD on 13 December 2021 with a history of rash for one day. The rash was associated with burning and itching. History of drug intake (tab fluconazole 150 mg) for tinea cruris one day back at 9 PM was followed by itching with rash at 2 AM at night. There was a history of similar lesions in the past due to some medication for a similar dermatological complaint. There was no history of fever or any medications. On cutaneous examination, well-defined erythematous plaques of varied sizes were present over the chest, back, lower limbs, and lips. Tablet fluconazole was stopped and tablet pheniramine 25 mg once a day for three days was started. Patient completely recovered from rash in five days.

Report the adverse event in the given SADRRF.

Version 1.4

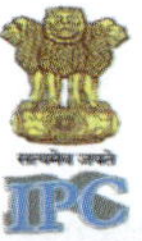

SUSPECTED ADVERSE DRUG REACTION REPORTING FORM

For **VOLUNTARY** reporting of ADRs by Healthcare Professionals

INDIAN PHARMACOPOEIA COMMISSION (National Coordination Centre-Pharmacovigilance Programme of India)

Ministry of Health & Family Welfare, Government of India, Sector-23, Raj Nagar, Ghaziabad-201002

PvPI Helpline (Toll Free) :1800-180-3024 (9:00 AM to 5:30 PM, Monday-Friday)

Initial Case ❑	Follow-up Case ❑

FOR AMC / NCC USE ONLY

Reg. No. / IPD No. / OPD No. / CR No. :

AMC Report No. :

Worldwide Unique No. :

A. PATIENT INFORMATION *

1. Patient Initials:	**2.** Age or date of birth:
3. Gender: M ❑ F ❑ Other ❑	**4.**Weight (in Kg.)

B. SUSPECTED ADVERSE REACTION *

5. Event / Reaction start date (dd/mm/yyyy)	
6. Event / Reaction stop date (dd/mm/yyyy)	

7. Describe Event/Reaction management with details , if any

12. Relevant investigations with dates :

13. Relevant medical / medication history (e.g. allergies, pregnancy, addiction, hepatic, renal dysfunction etc.)

14. Seriousness of the reaction : No❑ if Yes ❑ (*please tick anyone*)

❑Death (dd/mm/yyyy) ❑Congenital-anomaly
❑Life threatening ❑Disability
❑Hospitalization-Initial/Prolonged ❑Other Medically important

15. Outcome:

❑Recovered ❑Recovering ❑Not Recovered
❑Fatal ❑Recovered with sequelae ❑Unknown

C. SUSPECTED MEDICATION(S) *

S. No.	8. Name (Brand/ Generic)	Manufacturer (if known)	Batch No. / Lot No.	Expiry Date (if known)	Dose	Route	Frequency	Therapy Dates: Date Started	Therapy Dates: Date Stopped	Indication	Causality Assessment
i											
ii											
iii											
iv#											

9. Action taken after reaction (*please tick*)

10. Reaction reappeared after reintroduction of suspected medication (*please tick*)

S. No. as per C	Drug withdrawn	Dose increased	Dose reduced	Dose not changed	Not applicable	Unknown	Yes	No	Effect unknown	Dose (if re-introduced)
i										
ii										
iii										
iv										

11. Concomitant medical product including self-medication and herbal remedies with therapy dates (Exclude those used to treat reaction)

S. No.	Name (Brand / Generic)	Dose	Route	Frequency (OD, BD, etc.)	Therapy Dates: Date Started	Therapy Dates: Date Stopped	Indication
i							
ii							
iii#							

Additional Information :

D. REPORTER DETAILS *

16. Name & Address : ______________________________

____

Pin : ________ Email : ______________________

Contact No- : ______________________

Occupation : ______________________ Signature : ______________

17. Date of this report (dd/mm/yyyy) :

Signature and Name of Receiving Personnel :

Confidentiality : The patient's identity is held in strict confidence and protected to the fullest extent. Submission of a report does not constitute an admission that medical personnel or manufacturer or the product caused or contributed to the reaction. Submission of an ADR report does not have any legal implication on the reporter.

Use separate page for more information

* Mandatory Fields for suspected ADR Reporting Form

ADVICE ABOUT REPORTING

A. What to report?

All adverse events should be reported

Report non-serious, known or unknown, frequent or rare adverse drug reactions due to Medicines, Vaccines & Herbal Products.

Report every serious adverse drug reactions. A reaction is serious when the patient outcome is:

- Death
- Life-threatening
- Hospitalization (initial or prolonged)
- Disability (significant, persistent or permanent)
- Congenital anomaly
- Report intervention to prevent permanent impairment or damage

NOTE : Serious/Adverse Event following immunization can also be reported in Serious AEFI case Notification Form available on http://www.ipc.gov.in

B. Who can report?

All healthcare professionals (Clinicians, Dentists, Pharmacists and Nurse etc.) can report adverse drug reactions

C. Where to report?

Duly filled in Suspected Adverse Drug Reaction Reporting Form can be sent to the nearest Adverse Drug Reaction Monitoring Centre (AMC) or directly to the National Coordination Centre (NCC) for PvPI.

Call on Helpline (Toll Free) 1800 180 3024 to report ADRs or directly mail this filled form to pvpi.ipc@gov.in

A list of nationwide AMCs is available at : http://www.ipc.gov.in, http://www.ipc.gov.in/PvPI/pv_home.html

D. What happens to the submitted information?

- Information provided in this form is handled in strict confidence. The causality assessment is carried out at AMCs by using WHO-UMC scale. The analyzed forms are forwarded to the NCC-PvPI through ADR database. Finally the data is analyzed and forwarded to the Global Pharmacovigilance Database managed by WHO Uppsala Monitoring Centre in Sweden.
- The reports are periodically reviewed by the NCC-PvPI. The information generated on the basis of these reports helps in continuous assessment of the benefit-risk ratio of medicines.
- The Signal Review Panel of PvPI reviews the data and suggests any interventions that may be required.

E. Mandatory fields for suspected ADR Reporting Form (*)

Patient initials, age at onset of reaction, reaction term(s), date of onset of reaction, suspected medication(s) & reporter information.

For Adverse Drug Reaction Reporting Tools

- **E-mail :** pvpi.ipc@gov.in
- **PvPI Helpline (Toll Free) : 1800 180 3024** (9:00 AM to 5:30 PM, Monday-Friday)
- **ADR Mobile App : "ADRPvPI"**

NOTES

NOTES

CHAPTER 10 Oral Rehydration Salt Solution

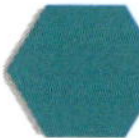

COMPETENCY

PH6.3: Devise pharmacotherapeutic plan to manage acute and chronic diarrhea in adults and children.

ORAL REHYDRATION SALT

Oral rehydration salt (ORS) solution is an oral powder containing a mixture of sodium chloride, potassium chloride, sodium citrate and glucose. After being dissolved in a required amount of water it is used for the prevention and treatment of dehydration.

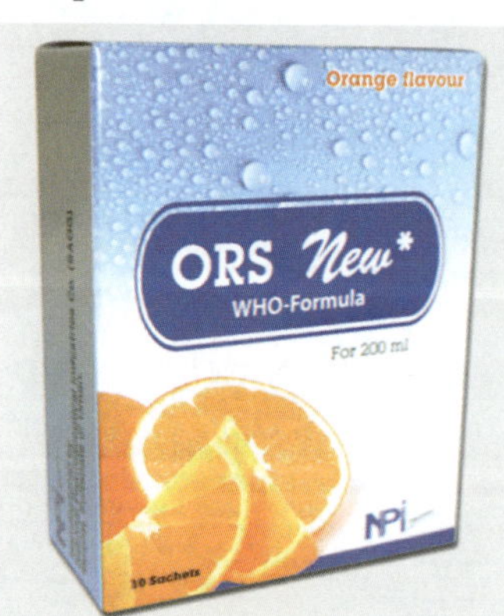

Composition-WHO New Formula ORS

Contents		*Concentration*	
Sodium chloride	2.6 g	Na^+	75 mM
Potassium chloride	1.5 g	K^+	20 mM
Trisodium citrate	2.9 g	Cl^-	65 mM
Glucose	13.5 g	Citrate	10 mM
Water	1 L	Glucose	75 mM
Total osmolarity			**245 mOsm/L**

Rationale for ORS Composition

- Solution should be isotonic or slightly hypotonic (200–310 mOsm/L) to be effective, as diarrheal fluids are isotonic with plasma, i.e., 290 mOsm/L.
- Apart from providing energy, glucose is also utilized in absorption of Na^+ from intestinal secretions. Thus, molar ratio of glucose should be equal to or higher than sodium, but not more than 110 mM.
- Sufficient potassium, bicarbonates and citrates should be supplemented for the losses in diarrheal fluids.

Method of Preparation

- Wash your hands with soap and water.
- Next, wash a container with soap and clean water.
- Pour 1 L of previously boiled and cooled clean water into the container.
- Add the ORS powder to the water, stir until all the powder has been mixed.
- Taste before giving it to the child, it should taste as tears, neither too sweet nor too salty.
- If it appears too sweet or salty, throw it away and prepare a new salt solution.

Homemade ORS

If ORS packets are not available:
- **Clean water:** 1 L - 5 cups full (each cup about 200 mL)
- **Sugar:** Six level teaspoons

- **Salt:** Half level teaspoon
- Stir the mixture till the sugar dissolves

Other Alternatives

Lemon juice with sugar, salt and water, butter milk with salt, coconut water can also be given.

Super ORS

- **Glycine fortified ORS:** It contains 20 g glycine amino acid added to WHO ORS. It reduces both volume and frequency of diarrhea but is more expensive.
- **Rice-based ORS**: It is a type of super ORS in which glucose is replaced with cooked rice powder or cooked rice water (50–80 g/L). It substantially reduces the rate of stool loss in acute diarrhea associated mainly with cholera.

Precautions to be Taken

- The prepared solution should be stored in a closed container and used within 24 hours of preparation. After 24 hours it should be discarded as solution contains glucose which is a good medium for bacterial growth.
- The prepared solution should not be reboiled.
- Strict hygiene should be maintained while administering ORS.
- ORS should not be used or if necessary, should be used cautiously in the cases of impaired renal function and intestinal obstruction.

Indication/use of ORS

ORS is used for the prevention and treatment of dehydration.

Causes of Dehydration

- Diarrhea (most common)
- Vomiting
- Heat stroke
- Excessive sweating
- Polyuria
- Diabetic coma

Zinc Supplementation with ORS

Addition of zinc along with ORS reduces both duration and severity of acute diarrhea in children less than 5 years of age. As per WHO recommendations and National Rural Health Mission of Government of India 10 mg (half tablet) is advisable to children up to 6 months and 20 mg (1 tablet) per day to children between 6 months to 5 years of age. The tablet is available as dispersible tablet that dissolves easily in a tablespoon of water.

Types of Dehydration

By clinical assessment it can be categorized into three types:

Observation	*Mild dehydration*	*Moderate dehydration*	*Severe dehydration*
Condition	Alert	Restlessness, irritable	Lethargy, sleepy/altered consciousness
Skin pinch	Skin goes back quickly	Goes back slowly	Goes back very slowly
Eyes	Normal	Sunken	Sunken
Tears	Present	Absent	Absent
Thirst	Normal	Thirsty	Not able to drink
Tongue and mouth	Moist	Dry	Very dry
Treatment	*Plan A*	*Plan B*	*Plan C*

Plan A

ORS is given orally

Age	*Quantity advised*
Up to 2 months	5 teaspoon after each loose stool
2 months to 2 years	50–100 mL (¼ to ½ glass) after each loose stool
2–10 years	100–200 mL (½ to ¼ glass) after each loose stool
More than 10 years	As much as child want

Note: If the child vomits, wait for 10 minutes and then restart giving ORS solution but more slowly than before.

Zinc Supplements for Children <5 Years of Age

- **2–6 months:** 10 mg (½ dispersible tablet) in breast milk in spoon
- **6 months to 5 years:** 20 mg (1 dispersible tablet) for 14 days with water

Plan B

- **Replacement therapy:** 75 mL/kg ORS is given in 4 hours
- **Maintenance therapy:**
  - Begins after disappearance of dehydration signs.
  - 10–20 mL/kg ORS is given after each stool.

Replacement therapy for children up to 5 years of age:

Age	<6 months	6–12 months	1–2 years	2–5 years
Weight	<6 kg	6–10 kg	10–12 kg	12–19 kg
Quantity of ORS	200–400 mL (1–2 glass)	400–700 mL (2–3 glass)	700–900 mL (3–4 glass)	900–1,400 mL (4–7 glass)

After 4 hours shift to Plan A—ORS with zinc supplementation

Plan C

Start intravenous fluids immediately.

- **Replacement therapy:** 100 mL/kg Ringer lactate IV fluid given intravenously
  - If age <1 year—30 mL/kg in first hour and 70 mL/kg in next 5 hours
  - If age >1 year—30 mL/kg in first half hour and 70 mL/kg in next 2 and half hour
- **Maintenance therapy:** Same as above.

Advantages of ORS

- Easy, simple and effective therapy
- Reduces dehydration and the need for hospitalization
- Low-cost treatment
- Treatment of patient at home is possible
- Does not require skilled person
- Effective for all age groups

EXERCISES

Exercise 1: Define super ORS. Enumerate its advantages.

Exercise 2: Why ORS solution should be discarded after 24 hours of its preparation?

Exercise 3: Write down the treatment plan for severe dehydration.

Exercise 4: Enumerate the advantages of ORS solution?

NOTES

CHAPTER 11

Prescription Writing

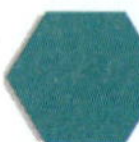

COMPETENCIES

PH10.4: Describe parts of a correct, rational and legible prescription and write rational prescriptions for the provided condition.
PH10.6: Perform a critical appraisal of a given prescription and suggest ways to improve it.

PRESCRIPTION

A prescription is a written instructions to a pharmacist and to a patient by a registered medical practitioner. Prescription should always be written in a legible handwriting and should always be complete.

Parts of Prescription

1. **Patient's information:** Name, age, sex, weight, address of the patient
2. **Prescriber's information:** Name, qualification, registration no., address, contact no.
3. Date
4. **Superscription:** It includes the symbol c. It is a symbol that stands for a Latin word "Take Thou" that means "you take". It is also considered as the symbol of the God of Healing - Jupiter.
5. **Inscription:** It is the main body of the prescription, and contains the names of medicines, dosage form, dose, duration and frequency. Drug's name should be written in UPPER CASE.
6. **Subscription:** This section includes instructions for the pharmacist on how the formulation has to be prepared and how many dose units are to be dispensed. In modern practice this part is somewhat modified as preformed drug formulations are available and the pharmacist dispenses them as per the duration and frequency mentioned.
7. **Transcription:** It includes instructions to the patient regarding drug administration, follow up visit, disease or health related advices. It is better to write instructions in vernacular language.
8. **Prescriber's signature:** This is the last but an important part and includes the signature of the registered medical practitioner. It is advisable to add the name of prescriber along with signature.

Additional Points to Remember

A prescription should also include the following points wherever relevant:
1. Relevant history—medical/past/occupation/travel/exposure/injury if any
2. Clinical reports
3. Relevant sign and symptoms, examination findings
4. Documentation of allergy/drug-related problem
5. Write medicines by their generic names
6. Write oral medicines first followed by injectables and then topical preparations
7. Put '0' before a decimal, e.g., write 0.5 mg in place of .5 mg
8. Write time gap between two doses, e.g., 6 hourly
9. Always mention maximum dose that can be taken in a day for drugs prescribed on 'as and when needed' basis

Avoid the Following Points in a Prescription

1. Avoid use of brand/proprietary names of medicines
2. Do not use whitener
3. Avoid abbreviations like PCM, CPM, etc.
4. NO '0' after decimal, e.g., write Insulin 2 unit in place of Insulin 2.0 unit
5. Avoid using Latin terms like AC, PC, etc.
6. Do not leave much space between the main body of the prescription and the signature

Record Keeping

- Inpatient records should be preserved for three years
- Outpatient records containing schedule H1 drug should be preserved for three years
- Outpatient records containing schedule 'X' drugs should be preserved for 2 years

EXERCISES

Exercise A

Comment on the given prescriptions and rewrite the correct prescription:

1. **Sushila**
   24 yrs Female

   Fever 2 days

   Rx
   Tab PCM 1 SOS

   Tab oflox-tz 1 BD X 5 days

   Cap Becosule 1 OD

....

....

....

....

....

....

....

....

2. **Suresh** **12/11/22**
15 yrs Male

C/O Diarrhea 2 days

Rx
ORS – 1 packet

Tab oflox-tz 1 BD X 5 days

Tab Sporlac –DS 1 BD

Cap Becosule 1 OD

....
....
....
....
....
....
....
....
....
....
....
....
....

3. **Kaluram**
25 yrs Male

Dr Rajesh Mathur
Reg No. RMC - 2931
10/12/22

Typhoid fever

Rx

Tab PCM	**1 tab 6 hourly**
Tab Cefixime–O	**200 mg 1 BD**
Tab Sporlac–DS	**1 BD**
Cap Becosule	**1 OD**

Follow up after 5 days

4. **Mevaram** **Dr Seema Sankhla**
30 yrs Male **10/12/22**

Diag - Malaria

Rx

Tab PCM	**1 tab 6 hourly × 3 days**
Tab CHQ	**600 mg after meals** **300 mg after 8 hours f/b** **300 mg BD × 1 day**
Tab Metris	**500 mg 1 tab 8 hourly** **× 3 days**

5. **Santosh** **Dr Anil Kumar**
50 yrs Male **15/12/22**

Rx

Tab Lisinopril	**20 mg 1 tab OD 7 days**
Tab Spironolactone	**100 mg 1BD**
Tab Omeprazole	**20 mg 1 tab OD**

Follow up after 7 days

Anil

....

....

....

....

....

....

....

....

....

....

....

....

....

Exercise B

Write a legible and complete prescription for the given condition with required instructions for the patient and communicate same to the patient in a simulated environment.

Exercise 1: A 46-year-old female Santosh Devi presented in Medicine OPD with complaint of morning headache for 1 month. On general examination, blood pressure was 150/90 mm Hg, pulse 76 per minute, rest normal. On her last month medical record, BP 130/90 mm Hg was mentioned. She was diagnosed with essential hypertension.

Write a legible and complete prescription for her.

Exercise 2: A 20-year-old male Suresh Kumar presented in OPD with complaint of rhinorrhea, dry cough and a feverish feeling for two days. On general examination, BP was 110/70 mm Hg, pulse 88 per minute, no fever, congestion in nose but no congestion in throat, chest examination was normal. Rest of the physical examination was normal. He was diagnosed with common cold.

Write a legible and complete prescription for him.

Exercise 3: A 50-year-old patient Rajesh Kumar presented in OPD with complaint of high-grade fever for 5 days, cough with yellowish sputum for 4 days, occasional chest pain and shortness of breath on exertion. On examination patient was febrile (temperature 102°F), tachypneic (respiratory rate 32/minute), chest examination showed dullness on percussion, bilateral rales and coarse crepitations. Chest X-ray revealed bilateral lobar consolidations. He was diagnosed with community acquired pneumonia.

Write a legible and complete prescription for him.

Exercise 4: A 25-year-old male patient Kalu Ram, resident of a slum area, presented with complaints of diarrhea for one week, associated with abdominal cramps and nausea. No complaint of fever, vomiting or passage of blood or mucous in stools. He has taken some drug for diarrhea from a pharmacy store, but not sure about the name. On examination abdomen was soft, no tenderness, rest was normal. A provisional diagnosis of amoebic dysentery was made.

Write a legible and complete prescription for him.

Exercise 5: A 45-year-old female Rajul presented with complaint of headache on left side, nausea and one episode of vomiting since morning. She was having difficulty in looking towards light. She revealed that she had such episodes in the past also and usually they subside on taking tablet ibuprofen. General physical examination was normal; BP was 110/70 mm Hg and pulse 80/minute. A diagnosis of mild migraine was made.

Write a legible and complete prescription for her.

Exercise 6: A 22-year-old male patient Raja Bhai presented in OPD with complaint of malaise, mild grade fever, cough with white sputum, anorexia and weight loss for 15 days. He revealed that fever is usually mild and starts in the evening. On general physical examination patient appears thinly built, afebrile and chest examination was normal. Chest X-ray revealed small unilateral infiltrates and hilar lymph node enlargement. Sputum examination showed acid fast bacilli. He was diagnosed with pulmonary tuberculosis.

Write a legible and complete prescription for him.

Exercise 7: A 52-year-old male patient Rajeev Kumar presented in OPD with complaints of pain and tightness in the chest after exertion like climbing stairs, for 2–3 months. The pain starts behind the sternum and radiates to left shoulder, is relieved after taking rest for some time. On examination BP was 130/80 mm Hg, pulse 78/minute, rest was normal. He is a known case of hypertension and is taking tablet Telmisartan 40 mg once a day. ECG at rest was normal, but exercise ECG showed horizontal ST segment depression that reversed when ischemia was relieved. A diagnosis of angina pectoris was made.

Write a legible and complete prescription for him.

Exercise 8: A 10-year-old boy Rohit presented in pediatrics OPD with his mother. He had complaints of watery diarrhea, bloating and nausea for one day. He passed stools 6–7 times on the previous day and had two episodes of vomiting. Physical examination was normal with no tenderness in abdomen. No history of fever, abdominal cramps or blood in stools. He gave history of consuming street food one day back. A diagnosis of acute diarrhea, probably of viral origin was considered.

Write a complete and legible prescription for him.

Exercise 9: A 30-year-old male Rajeev, a sales executive presented in medicine OPD with complaints of epigastric pain for 2–3 months. The pain is relieved by eating something bland, but reoccurs after 3–4 hours. He gave history of frequent intake of spicy food in restaurants due to busy schedule. General physical examination was normal. Patient was advised for upper GI endoscopy but he denied. A probable diagnosis of peptic ulcer was made.

Write a complete and legible prescription for him.

Exercise 10: An 18-year-old girl presents in OPD with complaint of severe itching all over the body for five days. She revealed that her brother and mother are also having a similar problem of itching. On examination marks of excoriation were present over both hands and abdomen, and small vesicular lesions were present on skin of hands, elbow, feet and abdomen. Small burrow like lesions were present on inter-digital spaces of both hands. No lesions were found on head and neck area. She was diagnosed with scabies.

Write a complete and legible prescription for him.

Exercise 11: A 45-year-old male Mr Rajesh presents with acute onset of severe pain, redness and swelling in the right first metatarsophalangeal joint. He has a history of similar episodes over the last 2 years. Serum uric acid level is 9.2 mg/dL. Joint aspiration confirms monosodium urate crystals. He has no known drug allergies and renal function is normal. He consumes alcohol occasionally and reports a high protein diet. A diagnosis of acute gouty arthritis with hyperuricemia was made.

Write a legible and complete prescription for him.

Exercise 12: A 16-year-old female Ms Khushi presents with multiple comedones, papules and pustules on her face and upper back. No signs of nodulocystic acne are present. She is otherwise healthy and has no history of allergies. She complaints of oily skin and occasional menstrual irregularities. She is not on any other medications. A diagnosis of acne vulgaris was made.

Write a legible and complete prescription for her.

Exercise 13: A 30-year-old nonpregnant female Mrs Anita presents with complaints of burning micturition for 2 days, increased frequency of urination and urgency, and lower abdominal discomfort. She has no fever, nausea or flank pain. Urine routine microscopy shows plenty of pus cells. Urine culture is awaited. She has no known drug allergies and is nondiabetic. A diagnosis of uncomplicated urinary tract infection was made.

Write a legible and complete prescription for her.

Exercise 14: A 25-year-old male Mr Rohit complaints of difficulty in falling asleep and staying asleep for the past 4 weeks. He reports of taking more than 30 minutes to fall asleep and waking up multiple times during the night. He has no history of hypertension, psychiatric disorders, no known drug allergies. He is a medical student and is preparing for exams, takes 3–4 cups of coffee daily and uses online study materials. A diagnosis of insomnia was made.

Write a legible and complete prescription for him.

Exercise 15: A 35-year-old female Mrs. Sunita Sharma, 55 kg weight, height 160 cm, complains of fatigue, pallor and shortness of breath on exertion for the past 3 weeks. She has no known drug allergies. She has history of menorrhagia for past 6 months. Her laboratory findings revealed Hb-8.0 g/dL, MCV-70fl, serum ferritin-10 ng/mL, serum iron-25 μg/dL, TIBC-450 μg/dL. A diagnosis of iron deficiency anemia was made.

Write a legible and complete prescription for her.

Exercise 16: A 20-year-old female Ms Kajal presents with a history of two episodes of tonic spasm of all muscles of the body over the past 6 months. Each episode lasted approximately 2–3 minutes, followed by confusion and sleep. Neurological examination is normal. MRI brain and EEG are suggestive of idiopathic generalized epilepsy. There is no history of head injury, substance abuse or family history of epilepsy. A diagnosis of idiopathic generalized tonic clonic epilepsy was made.

Write a legible and complete prescription.

Exercise 17: A 15-year-old male Mr Rohan presents with complaints of recurrent episodes of wheezing, shortness of breath and chest tightness, especially at night and early morning. He reports 3–4 episodes per week with nighttime symptoms twice a month. These symptoms are more frequent during winters. He uses a salbutamol inhaler occasionally for relief. Spirometry shows reversible airway obstruction. Based on GINA guidelines, the patient is classified as having mild persistent asthma.

Write a legible and complete prescription.

Exercise 18: A 28-year-old female Ms Lavanya presents with high grade intermittent fever, chills and rigors for the past 3 days. She has recently returned from a malaria endemic area in Odisha. On examination she has splenomegaly and mild jaundice. Rapid diagnostic test is positive for Pf antigen. Peripheral blood smears thick and thin confirms presence of *Plasmodium falciparum*. There is no evidence of severe malaria or complications.

Write a legible and complete prescription.

Exercise 19: A 10-year-old girl named Ayesha is brought to the dermatology OPD by her mother with complaints of intense itching on the scalp for the past 2 weeks, especially behind the ears and the nape of the neck. On examination live lice and nits are seen attached to the hair shafts. There is mild excoriation but no signs of secondary infection. No drug allergies are reported. Her mother also found lice in her sibling's scalp. A diagnosis of pediculosis capitis was made.

Write a legible and complete prescription.

Exercise 20: Satish, a 30-year-old male, was brought to the OPD by his wife, with hypopigmented patches on the skin, and complaints of loss of sensation in these areas. On examination, thickened peripheral nerves are seen and there is loss of power in limbs. A probable diagnosis of multibacillary (MB) leprosy was made.

Write a legible and complete prescription.

NOTES

NOTES

NOTES

NOTES

NOTES

CHAPTER

Prescription Audit

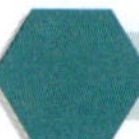

COMPETENCY

PH10.6: Perform a critical appraisal of a given prescription and suggest ways to improve it.

INTRODUCTION

- Prescription audit is a part of clinical audit and is a quality improvement process that is done to improve patient care and outcomes through a systematic review of care against clearly defined criteria and the implementation of change.
- It is a facility/institute level review exercise and should be conducted periodically.
- The purpose of prescription audit is to ensure that patients receive high quality care which is fair, cost effective and efficient.
- It is not a fault-finding exercise, rather a fact-finding exercise. It should be done in a transparent environment without any fear of punitive actions.

Prescription audit helps in assessment of:

- Extent of outpatient department (OPD) patient related information as recorded on prescriptions
- Prescribing habits of clinicians
- Appropriateness of medicine usage and its availability
- Drug dispensing practices and workload on dispensary

A good prescription should have the following details:

- Details of health facility—name, address, logo, contact number
- Details of the prescribing doctor—it should include name, contact number and registration number. As per government's directives, every prescription should have a seal/stamp that should contain doctor's name and registration number
- Details of the patient—name, age, sex, weight, address, contact number, beneficiary number (of health-related schemes)
- Clinical details:
  - Brief medical history including history of allergies
  - General physical examination: BP, pulse, temperature, chest, cardiovascular system (CVS), per abdomen and central nervous system (CNS) findings
  - Diagnosis/provisional diagnosis
  - Investigations
  - Prescriptions of medicines
  - Instructions for patients
  - Follow up details
- Signature

Electronic prescriptions are preferable. If electronic prescriptions are not available at the health facility, it is preferable to keep three copies of prescription. One is given to patient, second is for the pharmacist and the third should be kept for prescription audit.

Standard Treatment Guidelines (STG)

Institutional guidelines for treatment of common medical conditions help in better utilization of health resources and reduce irrational prescribing practices. National or state specific standard treatment guidelines can also be followed if institutional guidelines are not available.

Objectives of Prescription Audit

- To assess the extent of irrational prescribing
- Detection of prescribing errors with their reasons
- To reduce the irrational usage of antibiotics, syrups, injections, etc.
- To promote the practice of writing complete, legible and rational prescriptions by doctors
- To promote rational use of drugs
- Prescriptions of medicolegal cases should not be included in the prescription audit.
- The data should be analyzed and results should be reported. An action plan should be developed depending on the results and implemented to take forward the recommendations. It is a cyclical process that should be done periodically.

Sample size: Sample size a should be a representative of OPD attendance. For ease of calculation, a sample size calculator has been provided that has taken margin of error—10% and confidence level 95. Accordingly, 81 samples should be audited for OPD of 500, 88 samples for OPD of 1000, 94 samples for OPD of 3000, 95 for OPD of 5000 and 96 samples for OPD of 10,000 attendances, etc.

Prescribing Indicators

Indicators for Completeness of Prescriptions

Prescriptions should be assessed for completeness and scores should be given for each component and its correctness.

- Patient details—name, age, sex, address, reported allergy, date of consultation/registration in OPD date.
- Diagnosis or description of the health problem
- Medicine information—dosage forms, name of medicines prescribed in full or abbreviation, strength of formulation, dose, advisory (before/after food, at bedtime, etc.,) duration of therapy, medicine interactions
- Nonpharmacological treatment description
- Signature and information about the prescriber—doctor's name, qualification, registration no.

Indicators for Legibility and Rationality of Prescriptions

- Percentage of prescriptions with legible handwriting
- Percentage of prescriptions where medicines prescribed are in line with STG
- Percentage of prescriptions where allergies are mentioned
- Percentage of prescriptions with brief history written
- Percentage of prescriptions with provisional or final diagnosis
- Percentage of prescriptions where salient features of clinical examination are recorded
- Percentage of prescriptions where schedule/dosages are written
- Percentage of prescriptions with vitamins, tonics, or enzymes
- Percentage of prescriptions wherein antibiotics are prescribed as per Hospital Antibiotic Policy
- Percentage of prescriptions with prescribed injections

WHO Core Prescribing Indicators

Prescribing Indicators

- Average number of drugs per encounter
- Percentage of drugs prescribed by international nonproprietary name (INN)/generic name
- Percentage of encounters with an antibiotic prescribed
- Percentage of encounters with an injection prescribed
- Percentage of drugs prescribed from the essential medicine list or formulary

Patient Care Indicators

- Average consultation time
- Average dispensing time

- Percentage of drugs actually dispensed
- Percentage of drugs adequately labeled
- Patients' knowledge of correct dosage

Facility Indicators

- Availability of copy of essential medicine list or formulary
- Availability of key drugs

Format for Prescription Audit

As suggested by 'Prescription Audit Guidelines' document 2021 of National Health Systems Resource Centre, Govt. of India

Name of facility:
Month and year:
Sample size:

Sl. No.	*Criteria*	*Score in %*
1.	OPD registration number mentioned	
2.	Complete name of the patient is written	
3.	Age in years (≥5 in years) in case of <5 years (in months)	
4.	Weight in kg (only patients of pediatric age group)	
5.	Date of consultation—day/month/year	
6.	Gender of the patient	
7.	Handwriting is legible in capital letter	
8.	Brief history written	
9.	Allergy status mentioned	
10.	Salient features of clinical examination recorded	
11.	Presumptive/definitive diagnosis written	
12.	Medicines are prescribed by generic names	
13.	Medicines prescribed are in line with STG	
14.	Medicine schedule/doses clearly written	
15.	Duration of treatment written	
16.	Date of next visit (review) written	
17.	In case of referral, the relevant clinical details and reason for referral given	
18.	Follow-up advise and precautions (do's and don'ts) are recorded	
19.	Prescription duly signed (legibly)	
20.	Medicines prescribed are as per EML/formulary	
21.	Medicines advised are available in the dispensary	
22.	Vitamins, tonics or enzymes prescribed	
23.	Antibiotics prescribed	
24.	Antibiotics are prescribed as per facility's antibiotic policy	
25.	Investigations advised	
26.	Injections prescribed	
27.	Number of medicines prescribed	

Note: Each prescription is evaluated against above attributes in the form of observed response as 'YES' or 'NO'. In the end cumulative % is calculated for each attribute, e.g., % of prescriptions with antibiotics, % of prescriptions with injections prescribed, etc.

Source: 'Prescription Audit Guidelines' document 2021 of National Health Systems Resource Centre, Govt. of India. Available from URL: https://nhsrcindia.org/sites/default/files/2021–07/1534_Prescription%20Audit%20Guidelines16042021.pdf (accessed on 13/02/2023)

EXERCISES

Exercise 1: Perform and interpret critical appraisal of a given prescription.

Sl. No.	*Criteria*	*Yes/No*
1.	OPD registration number mentioned	
2.	Complete name of the patient is written	
3.	Age in years (≥5 in years) in case of <5 years (in months)	
4.	Weight in kg (only patients of pediatric age group)	
5.	Date of consultation—day/month/year	
6.	Gender of the patient	
7.	Handwriting is legible in capital letter	
8.	Brief history written	
9.	Allergy status mentioned	
10.	Salient features of clinical examination recorded	
11.	Presumptive/definitive diagnosis written	
12.	Medicines are prescribed by generic names	
13.	Medicines prescribed are in line with STG	
14.	Medicine schedule/doses clearly written	
15.	Duration of treatment written	
16.	Date of next visit (review) written	
17.	In case of referral, the relevant clinical details and reason for referral given	
18.	Follow-up advise and precautions (do's and don'ts) are recorded	
19.	Prescription duly signed (legibly)	
20.	Medicines prescribed are as per EML/formulary	
21.	Medicines advised are available in the dispensary	
22.	Vitamins, tonics or enzymes prescribed	
23.	Antibiotics prescribed	
24.	Antibiotics are prescribed as per facility's antibiotic policy	
25.	Investigations advised	
26.	Injections prescribed	
27.	Number of medicines prescribed	

Exercise 2: Perform and interpret critical appraisal of a given prescription.

Sl. No.	*Criteria*	*Yes/No*
1.	OPD registration number mentioned	
2.	Complete name of the patient is written	
3.	Age in years (≥5 in years) in case of <5 years (in months)	
4.	Weight in kg (only patients of pediatric age group)	
5.	Date of consultation-day/month/year	
6.	Gender of the patient	
7.	Handwriting is legible in capital letter	
8.	Brief history written	
9.	Allergy status mentioned	
10.	Salient features of clinical examination recorded	
11.	Presumptive/definitive diagnosis written	
12.	Medicines are prescribed by generic names	
13.	Medicines prescribed are in line with STG	
14.	Medicine schedule/doses clearly written	
15.	Duration of treatment written	
16.	Date of next visit (review) written	
17.	In case of referral, the relevant clinical details and reason for referral given	
18.	Follow-up advise and precautions (do's and don'ts) are recorded	
19.	Prescription duly signed (legibly)	
20.	Medicines prescribed are as per EML/formulary	
21.	Medicines advised are available in the dispensary	
22.	Vitamins, tonics or enzymes prescribed	
23.	Antibiotics prescribed	
24.	Antibiotics are prescribed as per facility's antibiotic policy	
25.	Investigations advised	
26.	Injections prescribed	
27.	Number of medicines prescribed	

Exercise 3: Perform and interpret critical appraisal of a given prescription.

Sl. No.	*Criteria*	*Yes/No*
1.	OPD registration number mentioned	
2.	Complete name of the patient is written	
3.	Age in years (≥5 in years) in case of <5 years (in months)	
4.	Weight in kg (only patients of paediatric age group)	
5.	Date of consultation—day/month/year	
6.	Gender of the patient	
7.	Handwriting is legible in capital letter	
8.	Brief history written	
9.	Allergy status mentioned	
10.	Salient features of clinical examination recorded	
11.	Presumptive/definitive diagnosis written	
12.	Medicines are prescribed by generic names	
13.	Medicines prescribed are in line with STG	
14.	Medicine schedule/doses clearly written	
15.	Duration of treatment written	
16.	Date of next visit (review) written	
17.	In case of referral, the relevant clinical details and reason for referral given	
18.	Follow-up advise and precautions (do's and don'ts) are recorded	
19.	Prescription duly signed (legibly)	
20.	Medicines prescribed are as per EML/formulary	
21.	Medicines advised are available in the dispensary	
22.	Vitamins, tonics or enzymes prescribed	
23.	Antibiotics prescribed	
24.	Antibiotics are prescribed as per facility's antibiotic policy	
25.	Investigations advised	
26.	Injections prescribed	
27.	Number of medicines prescribed	

NOTES

NOTES

CHAPTER

13

P-Drugs

COMPETENCY

PH10.3: To prepare and explain a list of P-drugs for a given case/condition.

P-DRUGS

P-drugs are personal drugs for the physician that has been chosen by him or her to prescribe regularly and the physician has become familiar with them. P-drugs are chosen on the basis of comparison of their efficacy, safety, suitability and cost. They are the priority choice for a given condition. P-drugs include not only the drugs but also their dosage form, dosage schedule and duration of treatment. P-drugs enable the prescriber to avoid repeated searches for a good and suitable drug in daily practice.

Every prescriber should have a P-drug list for common diseases and pathological conditions regularly encountered by him or her. It is also important to update and modify the P-drug list frequently with the help of available scientific literature. Before prescribing, it is important to justify the drug according to patient related factors, e.g., pregnancy, lactation, age, renal or hepatic status, etc.

Institutional, National and International Standard Treatment Guidelines are based on scientific evidence and consensus amongst experts. Therefore, they should be considered while choosing P-drugs.

WHO has published a practical manual on 'Guide to Good Prescribing' that defines the principles of P-drugs and how to choose them and prescribe.

The process of choosing a P-drug includes following steps:

1. **Patient problem:** The first step is to identify and define patient problem
2. **Therapeutic goal**: Specify the goal of treatment, e.g., cure or control of condition, prevention of complication, symptomatic relief, etc.
3. **Effective drug groups**
4. **Drug group (s) of choice** with justification
5. **Drug(s) of choice** with justification based on efficacy, safety, suitability and cost to the patient. Also choose appropriate dosage form, dosage schedule and duration of treatment.

After selecting P-drug for a patient, the next steps are:

1. Write down a complete and legible **prescription**.
2. **Communicate** the disease and drugs related information or instructions, any life style modifications required for the patient and the follow up plan.
3. **Monitor** the progress and continue or change or stop treatment accordingly.

So, practice of prescribing should be based on core principles of choosing and then giving treatment.

Example: A 20-year female Ramilabai, resident of Krishna Nagar, Udaipur, presented in outpatient department with complaint of fever with chills and rigors for two days. No associated complaint of burning micturition, cough and cold. Physical examination was normal. On PBF examination *Plasmodium vivax* was found.

Choose a list of P-drugs by following steps:

1. Therapeutic goal
2. Effective drug groups
3. Drug group of choice with reason
4. Drug of choice with reason
5. Write a complete and legible prescription

Solution:

1. **Therapeutic goal:**
   - Provide clinical cure
   - Treat symptoms
   - Prevent relapse
2. **Effective drug groups:**
   - For clinical cure of *P. vivax* malaria effective drug groups are divided into two categories on the basis of their erythrocytic schizontocidal action.
   - *High efficacy drugs:* Artemisinin compounds, chloroquine, amodiaquine, quinine, mefloquine, halofantrine, lumefantrine, atovaquone
   - *Low efficacy drugs:* Proguanil, pyrimethamine, tetracyclines, clindamycin, sulfonamides
3. **Drug group of choice:** High efficacy drugs are preferred due to reliable and fast effect. So, drug group of choice is 'High efficacy drugs.'
4. **Drug of choice with reason:** The patient is diagnosed with uncomplicated *P. vivax* malaria. As per National Vector Born Disease Control (NVBDC) guidelines, drug of choice for uncomplicated *P. vivax* malaria is chloroquine due to low prevalence of resistance against chloroquine in *P. vivax* in India. Artemisinin combination therapy is not preferred in uncomplicated *P. vivax* malaria for the risk of development of resistance.
   For treatment of symptoms paracetamol is added to treat fever.
5. **Prescription:**

Ramilabai Age: 20 years, Female Address: Krishna Nagar, Udaipur Diagnosis: *P. vivax* malaria	Dr Ramesh Kumar (MBBS, MD) Reg No.: 22134 Contact No.: 2204567210 Date: 1/1/2025

Rx

Tablet CHLOROQUINE 250 mg	4 tablets followed by 2 tablets after 8 hours 1 tablet twice a day for 2 days
Tablet PARACETAMOL 500 mg	8 hourly for 3 days

Take tablets with full glass of water
Follow up after 3 days

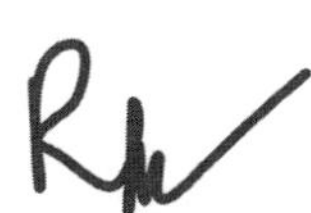

Dr Ramesh Kumar (Signature)

EXERCISES

Exercise 1: 28-year-old female Kanta Devi presented in OPD with complaint of high-grade fever with chills and rigors for one day. She also gave history of burning micturition and increased frequency of urination for three days. On general physical examination she was febrile, pulse 100/minute, rest findings were normal. Urine routine and microbiological examination reported bacteriuria and pus cells in urine.

Choose a list of P-drugs by following steps:

- Therapeutic goal
- Effective drug groups
- Drug group of choice with reason
- Drug of choice with reason
- Write a complete and legible prescription.

Exercise 2: A 23-year-old female Sulochana, six-month pregnant presents in OPD with complaints of easy fatiguability, breathlessness on exertion, palpitation and dizziness. General physical examination was suggestive of anemia. On investigation hemoglobin level was 8 g/dL and peripheral blood film was suggestive of hypochromic microcytic anemia.

Choose a list of P-drugs by following steps:

- Therapeutic goal
- Effective drug groups
- Drug group of choice with reason
- Drug of choice with reason
- Write a complete and legible prescription.

Exercise 3: A 48-year-old male Raj Kumar presents in OPD with complaints of generalized weakness and tiredness for last few weeks. He further revealed that he has increased frequency of micturition as well as increased thirst; he is on antihypertensive medication (for last five years) and has family history of diabetes. On general physical examination patient appears obese, blood pressure 130/90 mm Hg, pulse 80/minute, rest normal. He had with him previous month's fasting blood glucose report of 125 g/dL. On investigation, glucose tolerance test reported blood glucose 210 g/dL, HbA1c 6.7%, urine routine and microbiological examination was normal.

Choose a list of P-drugs by following steps:

- Therapeutic goal
- Effective drug groups
- Drug group of choice with reason
- Drug of choice with reason
- Write a complete and legible prescription.

NOTES

NOTES

CHAPTER 14

Drug Interactions

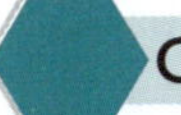

COMPETENCY

PH1.13: Identify and describe the management of drug interactions.

DRUG INTERACTION

It refers to modification in a drug's effect by another drug or food or beverage when they are administered together or in quick succession.

Drug interactions can be:
- Drug-drug interaction
- Drug-food interaction

The resultant modification can be:
- **Quantitative (more common)**: Response of a drug is either increased or decreased.
- **Qualitative:** An abnormal or different type of response is produced.

Drugs are often given together or in combination. Effects of one or more drugs can be altered by simultaneous administration of a drug or a supplement or even nutraceuticals. Drugs from alternative therapy systems like Ayurveda, Herbal, Unani, etc., can also interact with drugs from modern medicine system.

Drug interaction can be divided into two categories:
1. **Pharmacokinetics interactions:** These interactions alter the concentration of a drug or drugs at the site of action by affecting absorption, distribution, metabolism or excretion, e.g., ranitidine increases pH of gastric lumen and increases the absorption of triazolam, a basic drug.
2. **Pharmacodynamic interactions**: These interactions alter the response of one drug by another drug, e.g., aspirin, an antiplatelet drug when given with heparin, an anticoagulant, there is increased risk of bleeding.

The action may be increased, decreased or an abnormal response is produced. Thus, depending on the alteration, drug-drug interactions can be:
- **Additive**: When the combined effect is equal to the sum of the effect of each drug given alone
- **Synergistic**: When the combined effect is more than the sum of the effect of each drug given alone
- **Potentiation of toxicity**: Creation of a toxic effect from one drug due to presence of another drug
- **Antagonistic**: Interference of action of one drug by the action of another drug. Antagonism can be chemical, functional, dispositional or receptor mediated. Chemical antagonism occurs when two chemicals cancel each other's effect. Functional antagonism or physiological antagonism occurs when two drugs produce opposite effect on same physiological function. Dispositional antagonism occurs when one drug alters the disposition, i.e., absorption, distribution, metabolism or excretion of another drug. Receptor antagonism is blockade of effect of a drug by another, due to competition at receptor binding site.

Drug Interactions Before Administration

Some drugs when mixed in the same syringe or infusion bottle may interact and get inactivated. Some examples are:

- Ampicillin with gentamicin or other aminoglycosides
- Penicillin G with gentamicin or other aminoglycosides
- Thiopentone sodium with succinylcholine
- Thiopentone sodium with morphine
- Heparin with penicillin, gentamicin or hydrocortisone

Care should be taken that such drugs are not combined in same syringe or infusion bottle.

How to Prevent Drug-drug Interactions

- The doctor should have proper knowledge of possible drug-drug interactions.
- Take a proper drug history from patients including that of nonprescription drugs and complementary and alternative medicines.
- Record all the medications that the patient is taking before writing the drugs for presenting condition.
- Avoid polypharmacy.
- Suspect drug-drug interaction when a patient responds abnormally to any treatment.
- Be cautious when a hepatic enzyme inducer or enzyme inhibitor drug is prescribed with other drugs.
- Caution is also required when hepatic enzyme inducer or inhibitor is withdrawn.

Few Examples of Common Drug Interactions

Drug A	*Drug B*	*Reason of interaction*	*Result of interaction*
Salicylates (aspirin) *salicylates have high plasma protein binding, gastric irritant and antiplatelet effect	Phenytoin/methotrexate	Aspirin has high affinity towards plasma proteins, so displaces another drug	Toxicity of phenytoin/ methotrexate occurs
	Alcohol/corticosteroids	Both drugs are gastric irritant	Can cause gastritis and bleeding
	Probenecid	Inhibits tubular secretion of uric acid	Antagonize uricosuric action of probenecid
	Diuretics	Competition between both drugs for active transport in PCT and inhibiting PG synthesis by aspirin	Reduces or blunts diuretic effect
	Oral anticoagulant	Aspirin also have antiplatelet action	Enhanced anticoagulant activity so increased chances of bleeding.
Atropine *anticholinergic effect, delays gastric emptying	Antihistaminics/TCAs/SSRIs	All have anticholinergic effect	Additive effect
	Metoclopramide	Opposite effect on gastric emptying	Decreases prokinetic effect of metoclopramide
	Other drugs except digoxin, tetracyclines	Atropine delays gastric emptying	Absorption of most drugs is slowed but absorption of digoxin and tetracyclines increases due to longer transit time in gastrointestinal tract
Alcohol	Sedatives (narcotic analgesics, antihistaminics, TCAs, etc.)	Additive response	Increase CNS depression and motor impairment
	Disulfiram/metronidazole/ cefoperazone/sulfonylureas	Inhibition of aldehyde dehydrogenase by these drugs hence acetaldehyde accumulates	Aldehyde syndrome (disulfiram like reaction): Flushing, burning sensation, chest tightness, uneasiness, etc.
	Insulin and oral hypoglycemics	Acute alcohol ingestion depletes glycogen	Increase hypoglycemic effects
	Paracetamol	Chronic alcoholism induces enzyme which metabolize paracetamol to NABQI	Increase chances of toxicity even with 5 g taken in a day

Contd....

Contd....

Drug A	*Drug B*	*Reason of interaction*	*Result of interaction*
Phenobarbitone *enzyme inducer and sedative	Warfarin/theophylline/oral hypoglycemics	Phenobarbitone is an enzyme inducer	Decrease effect of these drugs
	Sedatives (narcotic analgesics, antihistaminics, TCAs, etc.)	Additive effect	Increase CNS depression and motor impairment
Levodopa	Carbidopa	Carbidopa inactivates peripheral decarboxylase enzyme	Increase effect of levodopa
	Metoclopramide	Metoclopramide crosses BBB and blocks dopaminergic receptor	Decrease effect of levodopa
	Pyridoxine	Pyridoxine activates peripheral decarboxylase	Decrease effect of levodopa
	MAO inhibitors	MAO inhibitors inhibit metabolism of peripherally synthesized DA and NA	Hypertensive crisis
	Antihypertensive drugs	Both cause postural hypotension	More chances of postural hypotension
Phenytoin	Rifampin/phenobarbitone (enzyme inducers)	Increases metabolism of phenytoin	Reduced effect of phenytoin
	Cimetidine/isoniazid/warfarin/ chloramphenicol (enzyme inhibitors)	Decrease metabolism of phenytoin	Increase blood level of phenytoin which can precipitate toxicity
	Sodium valproate	Decrease metabolism of phenytoin	Increase plasma level of free phenytoin
	Carbamazepine	Induce metabolism of each other as both are enzyme inducers	Decreased plasma level of both drugs
	Corticosteroids/theophylline/ oral contraceptives	Phenytoin is an enzyme inducer	Decreased effect/failure of oral contraceptives
	Sucralfate	Sucralfate binds with phenytoin and decreases its absorption	Decreases plasma concentration of phenytoin
MAO inhibitors	Cheese/beer/yeast extract	These substances contain large amount of tyramine which is not degraded in intestinal wall in presence of MAO inhibitors	Hypertensive crisis and cerebrovascular accidents
	Cough and cold remedies	These combinations contain sympathomimetic drugs. Interaction same as above	Hypertensive crisis and cerebrovascular accidents
	Pethidine	MAO inhibitors block hydrolysis but not demethylation, more norpethidine is formed which has excitatory effect	High fever, sweating, delirium, convulsions
Lithium	Furosemide/thiazide	Thiazide and thiazide like diuretics by causing Na^+ loss, promote proximal tubular reabsorption of Na^+ as well as that of Li^+	Increased plasma concentration of Li^+. Lithium is a narrow therapeutic index drug. It should be monitored as the drug interaction may leads to lithium toxicity
	Insulin and oral hypoglycemics	Lithium stimulates insulin secretion as well as increases peripheral glucose utilization	Risk of hypoglycemia

Contd....

Contd....

Drug A	*Drug B*	*Reason of interaction*	*Result of interaction*
Propranolol	Digitalis/verapamil/diltiazem	Additional depression of sinus node and AV conduction	Profound bradycardia and risk of cardiac arrest
	Insulin and oral hypoglycemics	Masking of the symptoms of hypoglycemia and delayed recovery from hypoglycemia	Risk of dangerous hypoglycemia
	Phenylephrine, ephedrine and other α agonists present in cold remedies	Blockade of beta 2 receptor mediated vasodilation and unopposed alpha receptor mediated increase in BP	Marked rise in BP
Sildenafil/tadalafil	Nitrates	Sildenafil is PDE inhibitor, potentiate action of nitrates	Severe hypotension
Quinidine	Diuretics	Quinidine cause K^+ channel blockade while diuretics cause hypokalemia	Increased risk of torsades-de-pointes
Oral anticoagulants	Broad-spectrum antibiotics	Broad-spectrum antibiotics inhibit gut flora that produce vitamin K	Enhanced anticoagulant effect and increased risk of bleeding
	Rifampin	Rifampin induces metabolism of warfarin	Decreased effect of oral anticoagulants
Corticosteroids	Oral hypoglycemic drugs	Corticosteroids cause hyperglycemia	Decreased effect of oral hypoglycemics
Erythromycin/ clarithromycin/ fluconazole/ itraconazole/ voriconazole	Warfarin/zidovudine/ cyclosporine/phenytoin/ sulfonylureas theophylline	Erythromycin and other drugs are inhibitor of CYP450 enzymes	Increased blood levels of drugs and risk of toxicity
Ciprofloxacin/ norfloxacin/ pefloxacin	Theophylline/warfarin	Fluoroquinolones inhibit hepatic drug metabolism	Increased blood levels of drugs and risk of toxicity

(TCAs: tricyclic antidepressants; SSRIs: selective serotonin reuptake inhibitors; NABQI: N-acetyl-p-benzoquinoneimine; CNS: central nervous system; MAOIs: monoamine oxidase inhibitors; DA: dopamine; NA: noradrenaline; BP: blood pressure; PDE: phosphodiesterase)

EXERCISES

Exercise 1: Enlist drugs that are hepatic enzyme inducer with the name of induced enzyme.

Exercise 2: Enlist drugs that are hepatic enzyme inhibitor with the name of inhibited enzyme.

Exercise 3: **A 35-year-old female Kusumlata was prescribed with following medicine for generalized tonic clonic seizures. She is a married woman and a mother of two children. Kusumlata is also taking oral contraceptive pills for preventing conception.**

Identify the possible risk of drug interaction in the given prescription with rationale.

Kusumlata **Dr Rajesh Mathur**
35 yr F **Reg No. RMC -2931**
10/12/22

Diagnosis: Generalized Tonic Clonic Epilepsy

Rx

Tab Phenytoin sodium 100 mg 1 tab 6 hourly

Follow up after 15 days

....
....
....
....
....
....
....
....
....
....
....
....
....

NOTES

NOTES

CHAPTER 15 Dose Calculation

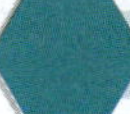

COMPETENCY

PH10.9: Calculate the dosage of drugs for an individual patient, including children, elderly, pregnant and lactating women and patients with renal or hepatic dysfunction.

DOSE

It is an appropriate amount of drug required to produce a desired degree of response in a patient, at a given time and can be repeated at an appropriate interval to produce a desired therapeutic effect.

POSOLOGY

The branch of science which deals with dose(s).

DOSE CALCULATION ACCORDING TO BODY WEIGHT

- ❖ Body weight influences the concentration of drug attainted at the site of action. The average adult dose refers to the dose for an individual of medium weight 70 kg.
- ❖ For exceptionally obese/lean individual and especially for children, dose can be calculated on body weight basis by using the formula:

Individual dose = (Body weight in kg ÷ 70) × average adult dose (Clark's formula)

If the dose is given in mg/kg/day and dose is required in mL:

- ❖ Calculate the dose in mg/day
- ❖ Divide the dose by frequency in a day
- ❖ Convert the dose from mg to mL

Example: Calculate the dose of ceftriaxone in mL for a child weighing 20 kg. Dose required is 100 mg/kg/day, to be given IV twice daily. The drug ampoule contains 40 mg/mL.

- ❖ Dose in mg/day = 100 × 20 = 2000 mg/day
- ❖ Divide the dose by frequency = 2000 ÷ 2 = 1000 mg per dose
- ❖ Convert dose in mL = 1000 ÷ 40 = 25 mL IV twice daily

DOSE CALCULATION ACCORDING TO AGE

- ❖ Pediatric dose = [Age ÷ (Age + 12)] × Recommended adult dose **(Young's rule)**
  Pediatric dosing according to Young's rule may result into subtherapeutic doses.
- ❖ Pediatric dose = [Age in years ÷ 20] × Recommended adult dose **(Dilling's formula)**
  Dilling's formula is used for calculating the dose for a child between 12 to 20 years of age.
- ❖ Pediatric dose = [Age in months ÷ 150] × Recommended adult dose **(Fried's formula)**
  Fried's formula is used for calculating the dose for a child up to 24 months of age.

Note: Dose calculations according to weight are preferred and used more commonly during clinical practice

DOSE CALCULATION ACCORDING TO BODY SURFACE AREA (BSA)

It has been argued that BSA provides a more accurate basis for dose calculation because total body water, ECF volume and metabolic activities are better paralleled with BSA.

Individual dose = (BSA in m^2 ÷ 1.7) × Average adult dose

BSA can be calculated by Dubois formula:

BSA (m^2) = BW (kg)$^{0.425}$ × Height (cm)$^{0.725}$ × 0.007184

It can also be obtained from chart-form or slide-rule Nomograms based on body weight and height. However, due to lack of data base and more cumbersome calculation, prescribing on BSA basis is done only for toxic drugs like anticancer drugs and a few other drugs.

For the rest of the drugs, body weight (BW) is used as an index.

EFFECT OF RENAL IMPAIRMENT

Plasma concentration and effect of drugs that are primarily eliminated by the kidney may be altered by renal impairment. Thus, in renal impairment, the dose of such drugs and nephrotoxic drugs should be modified according to the patient's actual glomerular filtration rate (GFR) or renal clearance. Example: aminoglycosides, vancomycin, amphotericin-B, cephalosporins, enoxaparin, allopurinol, atenolol, digoxin, etc.

Normal glomerular filtration rate (GFR) is 90–120 mL/minute/1.73 m^2.

For prescribing purpose on the basis of GFR renal impairment is categorized as:

- **Mild:** GFR 20–50 mL/minute and serum creatinine level 1.69–3.4 mg/dL
- **Moderate:** GFR 10 to 12 mL/minute and serum creatinine level 3.4–7.9 mg/dL
- **Severe:** GFR <10 mL/minute and serum creatinine level > 7.9 mg/dL

Note: Dose modification is usually not required at GFR > 50 mL/minute

Most commonly used formulae to calculate estimated creatinine clearance (eCrCl) or estimated GFR (eGFR) in renal impairment are:

1. Cockroft Gault formula:
   eCr Cl (mL/min) = {[(140–age) × weight] ÷ (72 × serum creatinine)} × 0.85 (if female)
2. CKD-EPI equation (chronic kidney disease epidemiology collaboration)
   $eGFR_{cr} = 142 \times \min(S_{cr}/k, 1)^{\alpha} \times \max(S_{cr}/k, 1)^{-1.200} \times 0.9938^{Age} \times 1.012$ [if female]

Where:

- S_{cr} = standardized serum creatinine in mg/dL
- k = 0.7 (females) or 0.9 (males)
- α = -0.241 (female) or -0.302 (male)
- $\min(S_{cr}/k, 1)$ is the minimum of S_{cr}/k or 1.0
- $\max(S_{cr}/k, 1)$ is the maximum of S_{cr}/k or 1.0
- Age–in years

Note: Online calculators are available for above calculations

Loading dose does not need modification in kidney disease as it depends on volume of distribution which is usually not altered.

Three types of modifications can be done in maintenance dose:

1. Decrease in the dose
2. Decrease in frequency (increase in inter-dose duration)
3. Both decrease in dose as well as frequency

TABLE 15.1: Dosing modifications of some common drugs in renal Impairment:

Drug	Normal dose	Dose adjustment needed (% of usual dose) GFR (mL/minute/1.73 m^2)		
		>50 mL/min	10–50 mL/min	<10/min
Enalapril	5–10 mg every 12 hour	100%	75–100%	50%
Atenolol	5–100 mg daily	100%	50%	25%
Thiazides	25–50 mg daily	100%	100%	Avoid
Furosemide	No dose adjustment needed			
Fluconazole	200–400 mg every 24 hours	100%	50%	50%
Cefixime	200 mg every 12 hours	100%	75%	50%
Ceftriaxone	No dose adjustment needed			
Clarithromycin	250 to 500 mg every 12 hours	100%	50–100%	50%
Azithromycin	No dose adjustment needed			
Erythromycin	No dose adjustment needed			
Amoxicillin	250–500 mg every 8 hours	Every 8 hour	8–12 hour	Every 24 hour
Ciprofloxacin	400–750 mg every 12 hours	100%	50–75%	50%
Ranitidine	150–300 mg daily	75%	50%	25%
Omeprazole	No dose adjustment needed			

Stock Solution

1% solution of any drug or chemical is known as stock solution. It is prepared by dissolving 1 gm solute in 100 mL solvent (10 mg in 1 mL).

- 1% or 1:100 = 1 gm in 100 mL
- 1:1,000 = 1 gm in 1,000 mL

TABLE 15.2: Lower concentration can be obtained by diluting stock solution.

Concentration	Strength	Content	Can also be written as
1%	1:100	1 gm/100 mL	10 mg/mL
0.1%	1:1,000	0.1 gm/100 mL	1 mg/mL
0.01%	1:10,000	0.01/100 mL	100 µg/mL

Unit

- Concentration of certain active biological substances or drugs is expressed in unit(s), e.g., insulin, heparin, etc.
- The unit is based on effect produced by a particular amount of drug in biological system.
- Example: 1 U is the amount of heparin that will prevent 1 mL of citrated sheep plasma from clotting for 1 hour after the addition of 0.2 mL of 1% $CaCl_2$ solution.
- Heparin is available in 40 unit/mL, 100 unit/mL, etc.
- One international unit of insulin is the amount of insulin required to lower the fasting blood sugar in a rabbit by 2.5 mmol/L

Some Useful Measurements

- 1 teaspoon (tsp) = 5 mL
- 1 tablespoon (tbsp) = 15 mL
- 1 pint (pt) = 0.47 L
- 1 cupful = 0.24 L
- 1 glass = 200 mL (approx.)
- 1 mL = 20 drops
- 1 mL = 60 micro drops

SUGGESTED READING

1. Munar MY, Singh H. Drug dosing adjustments in patients with chronic kidney disease. Am Fam Physician. 2007; 15;75(10):1487-96.
2. Kyriakopoulos C, Gupta V. Renal Failure Drug Dose Adjustments. [Updated 2022 Aug 8]. In: StatPearls [Internet]. Treasure Island (FL): StatPearls Publishing; 2022 Jan. Available from: https://www.ncbi.nlm.nih.gov/books/NBK560512/

EXERCISES

Exercise 1: Calculate the volume of ceftriaxone to be injected twice daily to a child suffering from meningitis when child's weight is 30 kg; dose required is 30 mg/kg/day and 4 mL ceftriaxone vial contains 1 g ceftriaxone.

Exercise 2: A child weighing 25 kg is suffering from pyrexia. Calculate the volume of paracetamol syrup to be given orally three times a day, when the dose is 30 mg/kg/day and the strength of paracetamol syrup is 125 mg/5 mL.

Exercise 3: Prepare a list of drugs that need dose modification in renal failure.

Exercise 4: Prepare a list of drugs that need dose modification in hepatic impairment.

Exercise 5: A child weighing 30 kg is suffering from chloroquine sensitive uncomplicated *P. vivax* malaria. Calculate dose and fill in the blanks given below.

1 tablet contains 150 mg of chloroquine base.

Dose	Schedule	No. of tablets
10 mg/kg	Start	....
5 mg/kg	After 8 hours	....
5 mg/kg	After 24 hours	....
5 mg/kg	After 48 hours	....

Exercise 6: A patient has been prescribed phenytoin 0.3 gram. How much volume should be administered to the patient if phenytoin is available as 125 mg/5 mL?

Exercise 7: How many vials of amoxicillin will be required to deliver 1 dose, if the patient's weight is 50 kg, dose of amoxicillin is 30 mg/kg/day, to be given in 3 equally divided doses and one vial contains 250 mg of amoxicillin.

Exercise 8: How many mg of noradrenalin is present in a 2 mL solution of strength 1:1000?

Exercise 9: How many mg of lignocaine is present in 10 mL ampoule of 2% lignocaine preparation?

Exercise 10: How many mg of adrenaline are present in a 10 mL ampoule. Adrenalin strength is 1:200000?

NOTES

NOTES

CHAPTER 16

Essential Medicine List

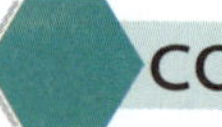

COMPETENCY

PH10.8: Describe Essential Medicines, Fixed Dose Combination, Over The Counter Drugs and explain steps to choose essential medicines.

ESSENTIAL MEDICINES

The WHO has defined essential medicines as "those that satisfy the priority healthcare needs of the population. They are intended to be available in functioning health systems at all times, in appropriate dosage forms, of assured quality, and at affordable prices for both individuals and health systems. They are selected with due regard to disease prevalence and public health relevance, scientific evidence on efficacy and safety, and cost considerations".

The WHO issued the first Model List of Essential Medicines in 1977, and since then it is updated every 2 to 4 years. The latest Model List of Essential Medicines was published in October 2021 by the WHO. It is a global concept that can be applied in any country, any individual healthcare facility, including both the public and private sectors. It is a dynamic document and is revised regularly according to changes in priority healthcare needs of the population.

The Ministry of Health and Family Welfare, Government of India, has released the latest National List of Essential Medicines (NLEM) in September 2022. The NLEM-2022 is given at the end of the manual.

Rationale for preparing an Essential Medicines List

- **Rational prescribing of medicines**: More experience with fewer drugs, nonavailability of irrational combinations, lower antibiotic resistance
- **Ensure quality of care**: Better quality assurance
- **Improved supply of medicines**: Easy procurement, storage and distribution
- **Reduction in healthcare cost**: Optimum utilization of healthcare resources and budget

WHO Criteria for Selection of Essential Medicines

- Pattern of prevalent diseases in the area
- Treatment facilities available at the center
- Training and experience of available personnel at the center
- Financial resources and affordability
- Genetic, demographic and environmental factors
- Adequate data on efficacy and safety available from clinical studies: International and National Standard Treatment Guidelines can help in selection
- Dosage form with ensured bioavailability and stability under available storage facility at center
- Cost comparison: Total cost of treatment should be considered, not only the unit cost of medicine
- Availability of storage facility
- Single compound should be preferred over fixed dose combinations (FDCs). FDCs are preferred only when the combination has proven advantage over single drugs given separately in terms of efficacy, safety or patient adherence.

Note: When two or more medicines appear to be similar in above respects, the choice between them should be done on the basis of relative efficacy, safety, cost and availability.

Additional Criteria for Selection as Mentioned by Selection Committee of NLEM 2022

- Licensed/approved by Drugs Controller General of India (DCGI)
- Aligned with the current treatment guidelines
- Recommended under National Health Programs of India
- Vaccines as and when are included in Universal Immunization Program

384 drugs under 27 therapeutic categories have been included in NLEM 2022. The medicines in NLEM have been categorized on the basis of level of healthcare system, i.e., Primary (P), Secondary (S) and Tertiary (T) level health care.

How to Prepare a List of Essential Medicines for a Primary Level Health care Facility

- Appoint a committee including all stakeholders, e.g., clinician, pharmacist, nursing person
- First of all, prepare a list of commonly encountered healthcare problems at the facility
- Enlist the conditions that could be treated at the facility itself considering the storage facility, specialized equipment and trained personnel available, e.g., diarrhea, worm infestation, malaria, typhoid, tuberculosis, mild to moderated hypertension, etc.
- Also include conditions where initial treatment is given before referral to higher centers.
- Prepare a list of medicines for above conditions from NLEM 2022 under Primary Level Healthcare category
- Consider National and State level Standard Treatment Guidelines
- Perform comparative cost analysis considering the total cost of treatment
- Prepare the final list of essential medicines
- Involve all stakeholders and circulate to all
- Keep on updating the document on regular basis

Fixed Dose Combinations (FDCs)

It is a combination of two or more drugs at a fixed ratio in a single dosage form. An example is cotrimoxazole which is a fixed dose combination of sulfamethoxazole and trimethoprim.

Advantages of Using FDCs

- Decrease in pill burden
- Increased patient compliance
- Cost effective

Above mentioned advantages are seen only when a rational FDC is used.

Disadvantages of Using FDC

- If an irrational FDC is used, it could result into decreased effectiveness of individual drugs and increased risk of adverse effects.
- In the year 2018 and 2019, a total of 405 irrational FDCs were banned in India by CDSCO.

Rationality for FDC

The rationality for any FDC is decided by following:

- The drugs in combination should act by different mechanism of action
- The pharmacokinetics of the drugs in combination should not differ significantly
- The combination should not result into supra-additive adverse effects

OTC Medicines

Over the counter (OTC) medicines are explained in chapter 20 (Dependence producing drugs and OTC medicines)

EXERCISES

Exercise 1: Considering yourself a member of selection committee, prepare a list of essential medicines for a rural primary level healthcare facility of your district, with the help of NLEM 2022.

Exercise 2: Enumerate a list of fixed dose combination medicines banned in last five years in India.

NOTES

CHAPTER 17

Drug Promotional Literature

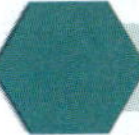

COMPETENCY

PH10.2: Perform a critical evaluation of the drug promotional literature and interpret the package insert information contained in the drug package.

DRUG PROMOTION

- As per WHO 'Drug Promotion' includes all the informational and persuasive activities by manufacturers and distributors, to induce the prescription, supply, purchase and/or use of medicinal drugs.
- All promotional claims should be reliable, accurate, informative, balanced and up-to-date.
- They should not include misleading or unverified statement.
- Financial or material gains should not be offered to or demanded by healthcare practitioners to influence their prescribing practices.

Based on WHO's ethical criteria for medicinal drug promotion, drug promotional literature should contain following information:

- Name(s) of active ingredient(s) using either international nonproprietary names (INN) or approved generic name of the drug
- Brand name
- Content of active ingredient(s) per dosage form or regimen
- Name of other ingredients known to cause problems
- Approved therapeutic uses
- Dosage form or regimen
- Side-effects and major adverse drug reactions
- Precautions, contraindications and warnings
- Major interactions
- Name and address of manufacturer or distributor
- Reference to scientific literature as appropriate

Apart from above mentioned criteria DPL should also be critically evaluated for exaggerated claims, catchy terms used, quality of paper and print, diagrams, tables and photographs given, statistical analysis mentioned, etc.

EXERCISES

Exercise 1: Critically evaluate the given DPL on the basis of WHO's criteria and comment.

Exercise 2: Critically evaluate the given DPL on the basis of WHO's criteria and comment.

Exercise 3: Critically evaluate the given DPL on the basis of WHO's criteria and comment.

NOTES

CHAPTER 18 Communication with Patients

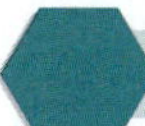

COMPETENCIES

PH10.14: Communicate with the patient regarding optimal use of a drug therapy using empathy and professionalism.
PH10.15: Describe methods to improve adherence to treatment and motivate patients with chronic diseases to adhere to the prescribed pharmacotherapy.

DOCTOR–PATIENT COMMUNICATION

The goal of Doctor–Patient Communication is to gather information to reach a diagnosis, prescribe treatment, provide instructions related to disease and treatment plan, and provide counseling when required.

Communication skills are those qualities which are used while receiving or providing information. Good communication skills help doctors in achieving patient satisfaction, better medication compliance as well as better clinical outcome.

Communication could be verbal, nonverbal, paraverbal and written.

Nonverbal Communication

It includes professional appearance, body language, eye contact, bedside manner, etc.

Paraverbal

Tone, pitch, accent of voice

Verbal Communication

While communicating with the patient following basic concepts should be followed:

- **Respect the patient**: Always respect the patient. It is better to use a language that they can easily understand.
  - Introduce yourself
  - Explain your role
  - Greet patient
  - Address with respectful words
  - Local language
  - Make the patient comfortable
- **Empathy**: It is the ability to understand and share the feelings of a fellow human being. A doctor should always have empathy towards his/her patients.
- **Active listening**: It means that while listening, the doctor should face towards the patient and appear attentive. His or her facial expressions should convey that he/she is concerned about the patient.
- **Use open-ended question**: Always start with open-ended questions like How is your health? What are your complaints?.....instead of close-ended questions like Do you have fever?
- **Cultural/racial sensitivity**: A doctor must always avoid using culturally or racially sensitive words or statements while dealing with patients.
- **Include the patient in decision making process.**

Difficult Situations

In clinical practice many a times communication with patient and relatives can be complex and difficult. Breaking bad news to the patient and relatives is a challenging task. It is important to understand the patient's perspectives and sharing information with them. Relationship building is important and helps in such situations. Communication with a violent patient or a psychiatric patient is another tricky situation that needs dealing with patience.

The **four basic principles of medical ethics** that should guide doctor-patient interaction are:

1. **Beneficence**: Always do good
2. **Nonmaleficence**: Never do any harm
3. **Autonomy**: Giving freedom to patient in choosing
4. **Justice**: Ensure fairness

ADVANTAGES OF GOOD DOCTOR–PATIENT COMMUNICATION

- Patient satisfaction
- Helpful in clinical practice
- Reduces risk of litigations
- Reduces mental stress on doctors
- Image building
- Increases job satisfaction

MEDICATION COMPLIANCE

It is the extent to which a patient follows the medical advice given by his/her doctor, e.g., dose, duration and frequency of prescribed drugs, lifestyle modifications.

Medication noncompliance is common amongst patients, especially in patients suffering with chronic diseases and elderly patients. In order to achieve a good health outcome, it is important that patient adheres to the drug regimen prescribed. General guidelines to improve medication compliance are as follows:

- **Simple regimen**: Keep the regimen as simple as possible. Polypharmacy and complex regimen decrease medication adherence.
- **Impart knowledge**: There are higher chances of compliance if the patient understands the importance of prescribed drugs and how to correctly take them. So, it is important to educate the patient in his/her local language, about instructions related to drug intake and precautions. Also, provide clear written instructions on the prescription paper. Avoid use of medical jargons and educate family members also, if required. Communication with patients should be tailored to their level of understanding.
- **Involve the patient in decision making** regarding the treatment strategy whenever possible.
- **Evaluate medication adherence**: The problem of medication noncompliance is many a times underestimated. So, it is important to check for adherence at the time of follow up visits. This could be done by asking direct questions related to drug intake or asking them to bring drug intake charts, empty blisters, etc.
- **Motivate and monitor medication adherence** on follow-up visits

EXERCISES

Exercise 1: You suspect medication noncompliance on a follow-up visit in a 45-year-old patient Meera Devi, suffering with type-2 diabetes. Enquire for medication nonadherence and counsel her for the same in a simulated environment.

Exercise 2: Communicate effectively in vernacular language, to a 30-year-old female patient about the proper use of tablet rifampicin.

Exercise 3: Communicate effectively in vernacular language, to a 30-year-old male patient about the proper use of enteric coated tablet of omeprazole.

Exercise 4: Communicate effectively in vernacular language, to a 40-year-old male patient about the proper use of liniment turpentine.

Exercise 5: Communicate effectively in vernacular language, to a mother about the proper use of ORS powder for her 2-year-old child suffering with diarrhea.

Exercise 6: Explain to a patient of pulmonary tuberculosis about the importance of medication compliance in a simulated environment.

NOTES

CHAPTER 19

Interaction with Pharmaceutical Representatives

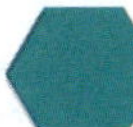

COMPETENCY

PH10.13: Demonstrate how to optimize interaction with pharmaceutical representative/media to get/disseminate authentic information on drugs.

INTRODUCTION

Doctors write prescriptions, so pharmaceutical industries try to persuade physicians to prescribe drugs from their brands. The most common method of one-on-one marketing is via the interaction of medical representatives (MR) or pharmaceutical sales representatives (PSR) with doctors. The medical representatives try to convince the doctors that their products are the best and should be prescribed in volumes.

The medical field is largely dependent on pharmaceutical companies for research and the availability of new drugs, devices, and diagnostic tests. Medical representatives also provide busy doctors with updated information on their drug products.

While interacting with MRs or other persons from the pharmaceutical industry following points should be considered:

- ❖ The doctors should be able to judge that promotional claims made by MRs are reliable, accurate, balanced, up-to-date and evidence based. MRs should not give unreliable and misleading information that might induce unjustifiable use of drugs.
- ❖ Doctors should confirm that MRs conveying promotional information have appropriate educational background and adequate training.
- ❖ It is also the responsibility of the doctors to confirm the claims made by promotional literature and MRs through valid scientific evidence.
- ❖ According to NMC guidelines while dealing with pharmaceutical industry, a doctor should always ensure that he or she should never compromise with his or her professional autonomy as well as the autonomy of his or her medical institute.
- ❖ A doctor shall not receive any gift, travel grant or personal favor from pharmaceutical industry of worth more than ₹ 1,000.
- ❖ A doctor shall not endorse any drug or medical product.
- ❖ Avoid meeting any MR during consultation hours. Avoid meeting MRs while patients are waiting.
- ❖ There should be a time limit fixed for meeting with MRs.
- ❖ MRs should not be given access to prescription records of patients.
- ❖ Free drug samples could be received by a registered medical practitioner and that may be provided to patients by the practitioner free of cost but not by MRs.
- ❖ A doctor should restrict him/herself in getting involved with promotional activities of Pharmaceutical Industries on social media platforms.
- ❖ Doctors should avoid using any company provided software where there is a risk of a leak of patient related data.

EXERCISES

Exercise 1: Mr Sushant is a medical representative. He meets Dr K Sharma for the promotion of a new drug formulation. Dr K told him that he will be attending an international conference after two months. Dr K asked him to arrange for his conference registration and travel.

Give your comments on above scenario.

Exercise 2: Dr A Singh is a busy practitioner. Mr S Kumar meets him in the OPD during evening hours. As there was a long queue of patients, Dr A asked Mr S to quickly brief him about his drug product. Mr S told him that the new drug formulation is the best antibiotic combination against gram positive infections. He further told him that there is no risk of serious adverse reactions as well as of resistance against it. He left a few free drug samples and drug promotional literature with Dr A.

Give your comments on above scenario.

NOTES

NOTES

CHAPTER 20 Dependence Producing Drugs and OTC Medicines

COMPETENCIES

PH10.16: Demonstrate an understanding of the caution in prescribing drugs likely to produce dependence and recommend the line of management.
PH10.17: Demonstrate ability to educate public and patients about various aspects of drug use including drug dependence and OTC drugs.
PH10.5: Identify and apply the legal and ethical regulation of prescribing drugs especially when prescribing for controlled drugs, off-label medicines, and prescribing for self, close family and friends.

DRUG DEPENDENCE

It is an altered physiological state that is produced by repeated administration of a drug in such a manner that continuous presence of drug in body system is required to maintain physiological equilibrium. Sudden withdrawal of such drug results into disturbance of physiological equilibrium, and that causes characteristic sign and symptoms collectively called 'withdrawal reactions.'

Drugs that are liable to alter mood and feelings are likely to produce dependence like CNS suppressants opioids, benzodiazepines, barbiturates, and alcohol. Stimulant drugs like amphetamine produce minimum or no dependence.

DRUG ADDICTION

It is a state where a person starts believing that his or her optimal wellbeing is achieved only through drug intake. It starts from liking the effects of drug and then progresses to compulsive drug intake. Drug addiction can be associated with both CNS depressant as well as CNS stimulant drugs.

DRUG ABUSE

It is self-medication of a drug in such a manner that is not approved by medical and social norms.

Misuse of some prescription drugs could result in dependence or even addiction. The most common drug groups liable for dependence are opioids and sedatives or hypnotics. Opioid analgesics are also mainstay for treatment of severe pain and are frequently required in palliative care.

CONTROLLED SUBSTANCES

Drugs or medicines that possess the potential for being misused or have a high risk of resulting into substance use disorder need to be controlled.

As per the Narcotic Drugs and Psychotropic Substances (NDPS) Order, 2013, the controlled substances are divided into three categories:

1. **Schedule A:** Manufacture, distribution, sale, purchase, possession, storage and consumption is subject to control. This schedule includes acetic anhydride, N-acetyl anthranilic acid, anthranilic acid, ephedrine and its salts, pseudoephedrine and its salts.

2. **Schedule B:** Export from India is subject to control. This schedule includes schedule A substances and ergometrine and its salts, ergotamine and its salts, iso safrole, lysergic acid and its salts, 3, 4-methylenedioxyphenyl-2-propanone, methyl ethyl ketone, norephedrine and its salts, 1-phenyl-2-propanone, phenylacetic acid and its salts, piperonal, potassium permanganate and safrole.
3. **Schedule C:** Import into India is subject to control. This schedule includes all substances included in schedule B except piperonal, potassium permanganate and safrole.

SELF-PRESCRIPTION

Use of prescription only medicines without the guidance or approval of a registered medical practitioner is considered self-prescription. While self-medication usually involves OTC medicines, self-prescription is more dangerous as it includes use of drugs which require prescription by a doctor. It could result into missed diagnoses, inadequate treatment and increased risk of adverse effects. Suggesting or offering prescription only medicines to friends or family members without consultation from a doctor is equally inappropriate and dangerous.

Steps to prevent misuse of prescription drugs:

1. Doctors should take drug history on every follow-up visit.
2. Obtain past history and family history of alcohol or drug abuse.
3. They should be suspicious of misuse or abuse when requirement of such drugs is increased or become more frequent.
4. Obtain a urine sample for investigation whenever in suspicion of drug abuse.
5. Give proper instructions to patients and also educate them about possible interaction of CNS depressant drugs with alcohol.
6. Patients should be instructed to never use other person's prescription drugs.
7. Patients should also be instructed to never stop or change a drug regimen without discussing with doctor.
8. Risk benefit assessment should be done before starting opioids. Start with lowest possible dose and then titrate. Taper the dose whenever possible.

Essential Narcotic Drugs (END)

Morphine, methadone, Codeine, Hydrocodone, Oxycodone, and Fentanyl are considered as ENDs by 2014 amendment of The NDPS Act (The Narcotic Drugs and Psychotropic Substances Act 1985).

Recognized Medical Institute (RMI)

Institute that fulfills RMI criteria can apply to state drug controller to procure and dispense ENDs. The authorization for RMI is only for 3 years, after which it should be renewed.

GUIDELINES FOR INDIVIDUAL REGISTERED MEDICAL PRACTITIONERS

Any individual Registered Medical Practitioner (RMP) may hold a small stock of following ENDs for emergency purposes in her/his own practice, without any special authorization:

1. **Morphine formulations:** Total quantity not more than 500 mg
2. **Codeine formulations:** Not more than 2000 mg
3. **Hydrocodone:** Total quantity not more than 320 mg
4. **Fentanyl:** Two transdermal patches one each of 12.5 μg/hour and 25 μg/hour
5. **Oxycodone:** Total quantity not more than 250 mg
6. **Methadone:** The upper limit of quantity is not mentioned in the rules

GUIDELINES FOR PRESCRIBING ESSENTIAL NARCOTIC DRUGS

1. Prescriptions must be in capital writing, dated and signed by the RMP with full name, address and her/his registration number.
2. Prescriptions must specify name, and the address of the person to whom prescription is given.
3. Prescriptions must mention the total quantity of the END, daily dose and the duration of the prescription.

Management of Prescription Drug Abuse

Diagnosis of prescription drug abuse could be confirmed by blood or urine test. Management depends on the type of drug, but counseling holds important role in all cases.

Counseling

Counseling of patients and family members by an addiction specialist could help in identifying the factors responsible for drug abuse, educating patients on how to resist cravings and prevent relapse.

Management of Withdrawal

Withdrawal could be dangerous and should always be done under observation and guidance of a healthcare professional:

- Withdrawal should be slow by gradual tapering of dose.
- Medicines that are used for opioid deaddiction are methadone, buprenorphine, naloxone and clonidine.
- No specific drugs are available for stimulant drug withdrawal.

OVER THE COUNTER (OTC) DRUGS

These are the drugs that could be purchased directly from pharmacy store without any prescription from a registered medical practitioner. OTC drugs are for common ailments like fever, pain, vomiting etc. Pharmacists play a major role in dealing with OTC medicines. As these drugs are taken without prescription, it becomes responsibility of pharmacists to provide instructions related to their use and possible interactions and adverse effects.

In India there are no specific regulations regarding OTC medicines, but medicines other than 'prescription only drugs (schedule H drugs)' could be procured as OTC drugs.

Common Concerns Regarding OTC Medicines

- Possible drug interaction
- Adverse drug effects
- Misuse especially of dependence producing drugs like analgesics, cough syrups
- Delayed diagnosis of underlying condition due to use of OTC drug, e.g., analgesics
- Incomplete information regarding precautions and contraindications on drug labels
- Sharing of medicines with other family members specially children without proper dosing information

EXERCISES

Exercise 1: You suspect analgesic drug abuse in a 21-year-old female. She visits your clinic frequently with nonspecific complaint of body aches. Physical examination and laboratory investigations show no abnormality. Counsel her about possible hazards of analgesic abuse.

NOTES

CHAPTER

21

AETCOM I: The Foundation of Bioethics

MODULE 2.2

At the end of the session, the student should be able to:

- ❖ Describe and discuss the role of nonmaleficence as a guiding principle in patient care (Level KH).
- ❖ Describe and discuss the role of autonomy and shared responsibility as a guiding principle in patient care (Level KH).
- ❖ Describe and discuss the role of beneficence of a guiding principle in patient care (Level KH).
- ❖ Describe and discuss the role of a physician in healthcare system (Level KH).
- ❖ Describe and discuss the role of justice as a guiding principle in patient care (Level KH).

Bioethics

Bioethics is the moral code of conduct that defines the right and wrong behavior in the practice of medicine, healthcare, research and biological sciences. A physician is expected to follow the principles of bioethics while interacting and treating his/her patients.

Basic Principles of Bioethics

1. **Beneficence:** The principle of beneficence states that the doctor must work for the benefit of patients and to promote the welfare of his/her patients. The doctor should always try to maximize the benefit and minimize the harm.
2. **Nonmaleficence:** This principle guides the doctor to work in such a way that he or she does not harm the patient. The physicians should weigh the benefits against the risks involved and work accordingly. If in certain situations there is no benefit to the patient, at least there should be no harm.
3. **Autonomy:** Every human being with a sound mind has the right to decide what should or should not be done with his/her body. According to this principle, the patient has a right to know the treatment options available, the possible benefit of any therapy or procedure and the possible risks involved. The patients should be a part of the decision-making process. Taking informed written consent from the patients is a part of the fundamental principle of autonomy. In certain situations, autonomy can be overridden, e.g., infants, children, psychiatric and unconscious patients.
4. **Justice:** This principle stands for fair and equitable treatment of every patient. It also includes equitable and appropriate distribution of healthcare resources. Sometimes priority is decided on the basis of need, severity and emergency of situation. But it should not depend on close acquaintance, favoritism or monetary benefits.

Ethics in Ancient India

Ethical principles related to professional and medical ethics have also been found in ancient scriptures. The best example is 'Charak Samhita', in which it is explained in detail that how a doctor should behave with patients and the ethical principles that should be followed by every healthcare professional.

EXERCISES

Exercise 1: Dr Arvind was a medical officer posted at a peripheral health centre (PHC). It was Monday and he was giving consultation to patients in his OPD. There was a long queue of patients outside even at 3:00 pm. His friend's mother visited the PHC for consultation. Dr Arvind allowed her to enter the OPD chamber for a check-up. Patients standing outside the chamber waiting for their turn did not like this gesture and resented it.

Discuss this case scenario with your classmates and write a note on the ethical principles involved.

Exercise 2: A newspaper has published a report that a doctor has removed the wrong kidney of a patient. The patient had the disease in her left kidney but her right kidney was operated and removed. Now she has lost her functioning kidney and is left with only one diseased kidney. She wants to sue the doctor in court.

Discuss this case scenario with your classmates and write a note on the ethical principles involved.

NOTES

NOTES

CHAPTER 22

AETCOM II: Healthcare as a Right

MODULE 2.3

At the end of the session the student should be able to:

- Describe and discuss the role of justice as a guiding principle in patient care (Level KH).

HEALTH AS A HUMAN RIGHT

- Every human life has an inherent dignity and that should always be preserved. Human rights have been universally declared by the United Nations Organization (UNO) on 10th December 1948. This declaration is known as the Universal Declaration of Human Rights (UDHR). This document contains 30 articles related to human rights.
- Article No. 3 states that every individual has the right to life, liberty and security.
- Article No. 25 states that every human being has a right to a standard of living adequate for the health and well-being of him/herself and of his/her family, including food, clothing, housing and medical care.
- Article No. 2 states that everyone is entitled to his/her human rights without any distinction of race/color/sex/religion/language/political opinion/nationality, etc.
- The above articles of UDHR clarify that every individual has a right to life with dignity and a right to health for him/herself as well as for his/her family. This right to health should be available to all without any form of distinction. These articles strengthen the fundamental ethical principle of 'Justice', which also states that medical care provided by a doctor should be fair and equitable.

HEALTHCARE SYSTEM

An ideal healthcare system of any country should provide quality healthcare services to its people and should be accessible, affordable and sustainable. The Indian healthcare system is a complex network involving government and private sector. The public sector consists of primary, secondary and tertiary healthcare services.

- **Primary healthcare services:** These are the primary point of contact and include primary health centers (PHCs), community health centers (CHCs), and subcenters.
- **Secondary healthcare services:** These include specialist services that are provided by district hospitals.
- **Tertiary healthcare services:** These refer to advanced services that include speciality and superspeciality services provided by medical colleges.

The private healthcare sector consists of corporate hospitals, nursing homes, clinics and individual practitioners.

Significant transformations have taken place in the last few years like the National Health Mission, the Ayushman Bharat Scheme, the Mukhyamantri Nishulk Dawa Yojana (MNDY), the Mukhyamantri Nishulk Jaanch Yojana (MNJY), etc. Despite these changes, the Indian healthcare system still faces many challenges like inadequate infrastructure, disparities between urban and rural services, a shortage of healthcare professionals, limited insurance coverage, etc.

SUGGESTED READING

1. The Universal Declaration of Human Rights. http://www.un.org/en/documents/udhr/
2. Kumar A. The Transformation of The Indian Healthcare System. Cureus. 2023;15(5):e39079. doi: 10.7759/cureus.39079. PMID: 37378105; PMCID: PMC10292032.

EXERCISE

Exercise 1: Write a note on the various healthcare schemes introduced in recent years that strengthen the fundamental bioethics principle of Justice.

NOTES

NOTES

CHAPTER

23 AETCOM III: Case Study on Bioethics

MODULE 2.5

At the end of the session the student should be able to:

- ❖ Identify, discuss and defend medicolegal, sociocultural and ethical issues as it pertains to patient autonomy, patient rights and shared responsibility in health care (Level KH).

INTRODUCTION

Bioethics is a moral code of conduct. It comes from within and is different from the rule of law. It is better learned in a group with group discussion. Learning with case scenarios and knowing the views of group members make the learning of bioethics more effective.

Case Study

A 21-year-old male patient Jagat has been diagnosed with advanced-stage cancer with a poor prognosis. Dr Jagdeep, the treating doctor has revealed this information to the parents. The parents of Jagat had an emotional breakdown after hearing the prognosis and requested the doctor to not reveal this information to Jagat. The doctor is now in a dilemma.

Discuss this case scenario with your classmates and answer the following questions:

1.1: Does the patient have a right to know the diagnosis?

____

____

____

____

____

____

1.2: Can family members request withholding of information from patient?

____

____

____

____

____

____

1.3: Whether the doctor should inform the patient about diagnosis and prognosis or not?

1.4: Write a note on the ethical principles involved in the given case scenario.

NOTES

Annexure

NATIONAL LIST OF ESSENTIAL MEDICINES–2022

	Medicine	*Level of healthcare*	*Dosage form(s) and strength(s)*
Section 1: Medicines used in Anesthesia			
1.1: General Anesthetics and Oxygen			
1.1.1	Halothane	S, T	Liquid for inhalation
1.1.2	Isoflurane	S, T	Liquid for inhalation
1.1.3	Ketamine	P, S, T	Injection 10 mg/mL, 50 mg/mL
1.1.4	Nitrous oxide	P, S, T	As licensed for medical purpose
1.1.5	Oxygen	P, S, T	As licensed for medical purpose
1.1.6	Propofol	P, S, T	Injection 10 mg/mL
1.1.7	Sevoflurane	S, T	Liquid for inhalation
1.1.8	Thiopentone	P, S, T	Powder for injection 0.5 g, 1 g
1.2: Local Anesthetics			
1.2.1	Bupivacaine	S, T	Injection 0.25%, 0.5% Injection 0.5% with 7.5% glucose
1.2.2	Lignocaine	P, S, T	Topical forms 2–5%, Injection 1%, 2%, 5% with 7.5% glucose
1.2.3	Lignocaine (A) + Adrenaline (B)	P, S, T	Injection 1% (A) + 1:200000 (5 μg/mL) (B) Injection 2% (A) + 1:200000 (5 μg/mL) (B)
1.3: Preoperative Medication and Sedation for Short-term Procedures			
1.3.1	Atropine	P, S, T	Injection 0.6 mg/mL
1.3.2	Glycopyrrolate	S, T	Injection 0.2 mg/mL
1.3.3	Midazolam	P, S, T	Tablet 7.5 mg; Nasal spray 0.5 mg, 1.25 mg; Injection 1 mg/mL, 5 mg/mL
1.3.4	Morphine	P, S, T	Injection 10 mg/mL, 15 mg/mL
1.4: Muscle Relaxants and Cholinesterase Inhibitors			
1.4.1	Atracurium	S, T	Injection 10 mg/mL
1.4.2	Baclofen	S, T	Tablet 5 mg, 10 mg, 20 mg
1.4.3	Neostigmine	S, T	Tablet 15 mg; Injection 0.5 mg/mL
1.4.4	Succinylcholine	S, T	Injection 50 mg/mL
1.4.5	Vecuronium	S, T	Powder for injection 4 mg, 10 mg
Section 2: Analgesics, Antipyretics, Nonsteroidal Anti-inflammatory Drugs (NSAIDs), Medicines used to Treat Gout and Disease Modifying Agents used in Rheumatoid Disorders			
2.1: Non-opioid Analgesics, Antipyretics and Nonsteroidal Anti-inflammatory Drugs			
2.1.1	Acetylsalicylic acid	P, S, T	Tablet 300 mg to 500 mg (effervescent/dispersible/enteric coated tablet 300 mg to 500 mg)

	Medicine	*Level of healthcare*	*Dosage form(s) and strength(s)*
2.1.2	Diclofenac	P, S, T	Tablet 50 mg; Injection 25 mg/mL
2.1.3	Ibuprofen	P, S, T	Tablet 200 mg, 400 mg; Oral liquid 100 mg/5 mL (p)
2.1.4	Mefenamic acid	P, S, T	Tablet 250 mg; Oral liquid 100 mg/5 mL (p)
2.1.5	Paracetamol	P, S, T	Tablet 500 mg, 650 mg Oral liquid 120 mg/5 mL (p),125 mg/5 mL, 250 mg/5 mL (p); Injection 150 mg/mL; Suppository 80 mg, 170 mg
2.2: Opioid Analgesics			
2.2.1	Fentanyl	S, T	Injection 50 µg/mL
2.2.2	Morphine	P, S, T	Tablet 10 mg; Injection 10 mg/mL, 15 mg/mL
2.2.3	Tramadol	S, T	Capsule 50 mg, 100 mg; Injection 50 mg/mL
2.3: Medicines used to Treat Gout			
2.3.1	Allopurinol	P, S, T	Tablet 100 mg, 300 mg
2.3.2	Colchicine	P, S, T	Tablet 0.5 mg
2.4: Disease Modifying Agents used in Rheumatoid Disorders			
2.4.1	Azathioprine	S, T	Tablet 25 mg (p), 50 mg
2.4.2	Hydroxychloroquine	P, S, T	Tablet 200 mg, 400 mg
2.4.3	Methotrexate	P, S, T	Tablet 2.5 mg, 5 mg,10 mg
2.4.4	Sulfasalazine	S, T	Tablet 500 mg
Section 3: Antiallergics and Medicines used in Anaphylaxis			
3.1	Adrenaline	P, S, T	Injection 1 mg/mL
3.2	Cetirizine	P, S, T	Tablet 10 mg; Oral liquid 5 mg/5 mL (p)
3.3	Dexamethasone	P, S, T	Tablet 0.5 mg, 2 mg, 4 mg; Oral liquid 0.5 mg/5 mL (p); Injection 4 mg/mL
3.4	Hydrocortisone	P, S, T	Tablet 5 mg,10 mg; Powder for injection 100 mg, 200 mg
3.5	Pheniramine	P, S, T	Injection 22.75 mg/mL
3.6	Prednisolone	P, S, T	Tablet 5 mg, 10 mg, 20 mg; Oral liquid 5 mg/5 mL (p), 15 mg/5 mL (p)
Section 4: Antidotes and Other Substances used in Management of Poisonings/Envenomation			
4.1: Nonspecific			
4.1.1	Activated charcoal	P, S, T	Powder (as licensed)
4.2: Specific			
4.2.1	Atropine	P, S, T	Injection 0.6 mg/mL
4.2.2	Calcium gluconate	P, S, T	Injection 100 mg/mL
4.2.3	D- Penicillamine	P, S, T	Capsule 150 mg (p), 250 mg
4.2.4	Desferrioxamine	S, T	Powder for injection 500 mg
4.2.5	Methylthioninium chloride (methylene blue)	S, T	Injection 10 mg/mL
4.2.6	N-acetylcysteine	P, S, T	Sachet 200 mg; Injection 200 mg/mL
4.2.7	Naloxone	P, S, T	Injection 0.4 mg/mL
4.2.8	Neostigmine	P, S, T	Injection 0.5 mg/mL
4.2.9	Pralidoxime chloride (2-PAM)	P, S, T	Injection 25 mg/mL
4.2.10	Snake venom antiserum	P, S, T	Soluble/liquid polyvalent (as licensed) Lyophilized polyvalent (as licensed)

	Medicine	Level of healthcare	Dosage form(s) and strength(s)
4.2.11	Sodium nitrite	S, T	Injection 30 mg/mL
4.2.12	Sodium thiosulfate	S, T	Injection 250 mg/mL
Section 5: Medicines used in Neurological Disorders			
5.1: Anticonvulsants/Antiepileptics			
5.1.1	Carbamazepine	P, S, T	Tablet 100 mg, 200 mg, 400 mg Modified release tablet 200 mg, 400 mg Oral liquid 100 mg/5 mL (p)
5.1.2	Clobazam	S, T	Tablet 5 mg, 10 mg
5.1.3	Diazepam	P, S, T	Oral liquid 2 mg/5 mL (p); Injection 5 mg/mL; Suppository 5 mg
5.1.4	Levetiracetam	S, T	Tablet 250 mg, 500 mg, 750 mg Modified release tablet 750 mg; Oral liquid 100 mg/mL (p); Injection 100 mg/mL
5.1.5	Lorazepam	P, S, T	Tablet 1 mg, 2 mg; Injection 2 mg/mL, 4 mg/mL
5.1.6	Magnesium sulfate	S, T	Injection 500 mg/mL
5.1.7	Midazolam	P, S, T	Tablet 7.5 mg, 15 mg; Nasal spray 0.5 mg/actuation, 1.25 mg/actuation; Injection 1 mg/mL, 5 mg/mL
5.1.8	Phenobarbitone	P, S, T	Tablet 30 mg, 60 mg; Oral liquid 20 mg/5 mL (p)
		S, T	Injection 200 mg/mL
5.1.9	Phenytoin	P, S, T	Tablet 50 mg, 100 mg, 300 mg; Modified-release tablet 300 mg; Oral liquid 30 mg/5 mL (p), 125 mg/5 mL (p); Injection 25 mg/mL, 50 mg/mL
5.1.10	Sodium valproate	P, S, T	Tablet 200 mg, 300 mg, 500 mg; Modified release tablet 300 mg, 500 mg; Oral liquid 200 mg/5 mL (p)
		S, T	Injection 100 mg/mL
5.2: Antimigraine Medicines			
5.2.1	Acetylsalicylic acid	P, S, T	Tablet 300 mg to 500 mg (effervescent/dispersible/enteric coated tablet 300 mg to 500 mg)
5.2.2	Ibuprofen	P, S, T	Tablet 200 mg, 400 mg; Oral liquid 100 mg/5 mL (p)
5.2.3	Paracetamol	P, S, T	Tablet 500 mg, 650 mg; Oral liquid 120 mg/5 mL (p),125 mg/5 mL (p), 250 mg/5 mL (p)
5.2.4	Sumatriptan	P, S, T	Tablet 25 mg, 50 mg
5.2.1: For Prophylaxis			
5.2.1.1	Amitriptyline	P, S, T	Tablet 10 mg, 25 mg, 75 mg
5.2.1.2	Flunarizine	P, S, T	Tablet 5 mg, 10 mg
5.2.1.3	Propranolol	P, S, T	Tablet 10 mg, 20 mg, 40 mg
5.3: Antiparkinsonism Medicines			
5.3.1	Levodopa (A) + Carbidopa (B)	P, S, T	Tablets 100 mg (A) + 10 mg (B), 100 mg (A) + 25 mg (B), 250 mg (A) + 25 mg (B); Modified-release tablet 100 mg (A) + 25 mg (B), 200 mg (A) + 50 mg (B)
5.3.2	Trihexyphenidyl	P, S, T	Tablet 2 mg
5.4: Medicines used in Dementia			
5.4.1	Donepezil	S, T	Tablet 5 mg, 10 mg

	Medicine	Level of healthcare	Dosage form(s) and strength(s)
Section 6: Anti-infective Medicines			
6.1: Anthelminthics			
6.1.1: Intestinal Anthelminthics			
6.1.1.1	Albendazole	P, S, T	Tablet 400 mg, Chewable tablet 400 mg; Oral liquid 200 mg/5 mL (p)
6.1.1.2	Mebendazole	P, S, T	Tablet 100 mg; Oral liquid 100 mg/5 mL (p)
6.1.2: Antifilarial			
6.1.2.1	Albendazole	P, S, T	Tablet 400 mg, Chewable Tablet 400 mg; Oral liquid 200 mg/5 mL (p)
6.1.2.2	Diethylcarbamazine (DEC)	P, S, T	Tablet 50 mg, 100 mg; Oral liquid 120 mg/5 mL (p)
6.1.2.3	Ivermectin	P, S, T	Tablet 6 mg, 12 mg
6.1.3: Antischistosomal and Antitrematodal Medicine			
6.1.3.1	Praziquantel	S, T	Tablet 600 mg
6.2: Antibacterials			
6.2.1	**Beta-lactam Medicines**		
6.2.1.1	Amoxicillin	P, S, T	Capsule 250 mg, 500 mg; Oral liquid 125 mg/5 mL (p), 250 mg/5 mL (p); Powder for injection 250 mg, 500 mg, 1000 mg
6.2.1.2	Amoxicillin (A) + Clavulanic acid (B)	P, S, T	Tablet 500 mg (A) + 125 mg (B); Oral liquid 200 mg (A) + 28.5 mg (B)/5 mL (p) Dry syrup 125 mg (A) + 31.25 (B)/5 mL (p)
		S, T	Powder for injection 500 mg (A) + 100 mg (B) Powder for injection 1 g (A) + 200 mg (B)
6.2.1.3	Ampicillin	P, S, T	Powder for Injection 500 mg, 1000 mg
6.2.1.4	Benzathine benzylpenicillin	P, S, T	Powder for injection 6 lac units, 12 lac units, 24 lac units
6.2.1.5	Benzylpenicillin	P, S, T	Powder for injection 5 lac units, 10 lac units
6.2.1.6	Cefadroxil	P, S, T	Tablet 500 mg, 100 mg; Oral liquid 125 mg/5 mL (p)
6.2.1.7	Cefazolin	P, S, T	Powder for injection 500 mg, 1000 mg
6.2.1.8	Cefixime	S, T	Tablet 200 mg, 400 mg; Oral liquid 50 mg/5 mL (p), 100 mg/5 mL (p)
6.2.1.9	Cefotaxime	S, T	Powder for injection 250 mg, 500 mg,1000 mg
6.2.1.10	Ceftazidime	S, T	Powder for injection 250 mg,1000 mg
6.2.1.11	Ceftriaxone	S, T	Powder for injection 250 mg, 500 mg, 1000 mg, 2000 mg
6.2.1.12	Cloxacillin	P, S, T	Capsule 250 mg, 500 mg; Oral liquid 125 mg/5 mL (p); Powder for injection 250 mg
6.2.1.13	Piperacillin (A) + Tazobactam (B)	T	Powder for injection 1000 mg (A) + 125 mg (B), 2000 mg (A) + 250 mg (B), 4000 mg (A) + 500 mg (B)
6.2.1.14	Meropenem	T	Powder for Injection 500 mg (as trihydrate), 1000 mg (as trihydrate)
6.2.2: Other Antibacterials			
6.2.2.1	Azithromycin	P, S, T	Tablet 250 mg, 500 mg; Oral liquid 200 mg/5 mL (p); Powder for injection 500 mg
6.2.2.2	Cefuroxime	P, S, T	Tablet 500 mg; Oral liquid 125 mg/5 mL (p); Injection 1500 mg
6.2.2.3	Ciprofloxacin	P, S, T	Tablet 250 mg, 500 mg; Oral liquid 250 mg/5 mL (p); Injection 200 mg/100 mL
6.2.2.4	Clarithromycin	S, T	Tablet 250 mg, 500 mg; Oral liquid 125 mg/5 mL (p)
6.2.2.5	Clindamycin	P, S, T	Capsule 150 mg, 300 mg; Injection 150 mg/mL

	Medicine	*Level of healthcare*	*Dosage form(s) and strength(s)*
6.2.2.6	Co-trimoxazole [Sulphamethoxazole (A) + Trimethoprim (B)]	P, S, T	Tablet 400 mg (A) + 80 mg (B), 800 mg (A) + 160 mg (B); Oral liquid 200 mg (A) + 40 mg (B)/5 mL (p)
6.2.2.7	Doxycycline	P, S, T	Capsule 100 mg; Dry syrup 50 mg/5 mL (p); Power for injection 100 mg
6.2.2.8	Gentamicin	P, S, T	Injection 10 mg/mL, 40 mg/mL
6.2.2.9	Metronidazole	P, S, T	Tablet 200 mg, 400 mg; Oral liquid 200 mg/5 mL (p); Injection 500 mg/100 mL
6.2.2.10	Nitrofurantoin	P, S, T	Tablet 100 mg; Oral liquid 25 mg/5 mL (p)
6.2.2.11	Phenoxymethyl penicillin	P, S, T	Tablet 250 mg
6.2.2.12	Procaine benzylpenicillin	P, S, T	Powder for injection 1000 mg (= 1 million IU)
6.2.2.13	Vancomycin	S, T	Capsule 125 mg, 250 mg; Powder for injection 250 mg,500 mg,1000 mg
6.3: Antileprosy Medicines			
6.3.1	Clofazimine	P, S, T	Capsule 50 mg, 100 mg
6.3.2	Dapsone	P, S, T	Tablet 50 mg, 100 mg
6.3.3	Rifampicin	P, S, T	Capsule 150 mg, 300 mg
6.4: Antituberculosis Medicines			
6.4.1	Amikacin	S, T	Injection 100 mg/mL, 250 mg/mL, 500 mg/mL
6.4.2	Bedaquiline	T	Tablet 100 mg
6.4.3	Clarithromycin	S, T	Tablet 250 mg, 500 mg, 750 mg
6.4.4	Clofazimine	S, T	Capsule 50 mg, 100 mg
6.4.5	Cycloserine	S, T	Capsule 125 mg, 250 mg
6.4.6	Delamanid	T	Tablet 50 mg
6.4.7	Ethambutol	P, S, T	Tablet 200 mg, 400 mg, 600 mg,800 mg
6.4.8	Ethionamide	S, T	Tablet 125 mg, 250 mg
6.4.9	Isoniazid	P, S, T	Tablet 100 mg, 300 mg; Oral liquid 50 mg/5 mL (p)
6.4.10	Levofloxacin	P, S, T	Tablet 250 mg, 500 mg, 750 mg
6.4.11	Linezolid	P, S, T	Tablet 300 mg, 600 mg
6.4.12	Moxifloxacin	P, S, T	Tablet 400 mg
6.4.13	Para- aminosalicylic acid	S, T	Granules (as licensed)
6.4.14	Pyrazinamide	P, S, T	Tablet 500 mg, 750 mg, 1000 mg,1500 mg; Oral liquid 250 mg/5 mL (p)
6.4.15	Rifampicin	P, S, T	Capsule 150 mg, 300 mg, 450 mg, 600 mg; Oral liquid 100 mg/5 mL (p)
6.4.16	Streptomycin	P, S, T	Powder for injection 750 mg, 1000 mg
6.5: Antifungal Medicines			
6.5.1	Amphotericin B	S, T	Amphotericin B (conventional): Injection 50 mg/vial Lipid amphotericin B: Injection 50 mg/vial Liposomal amphotericin B: Injection 50 mg/vial
6.5.2	Clotrimazole	P, S, T	Pessary 100 mg
6.5.3	Fluconazole	P, S, T	Tablet 50 mg, 100 mg, 50 mg, 200 mg, 400 mg; Oral liquid 50 mg/5 mL (p)
		S, T	Injection 200 mg/100 mL
6.5.4	Griseofulvin	P, S, T	Tablet 125 mg, 250 mg, 375 mg
6.5.5	Itraconazole	S, T	Capsule 100 mg, 200 mg; Oral liquid 10 mg/mL

	Medicine	*Level of healthcare*	*Dosage form(s) and strength(s)*
6.5.6	Mupirocin	P, S, T	Ointment 2%
6.5.7	Nystatin	S, T	Pessary 1 Lac IU, Oral liquid 1 Lac IU/mL (p)
6.5.8	Terbinafine	P, S, T	Cream 1%
6.6: Antiviral Medicines			
6.6.1: Antiherpes Medicines			
6.6.1.1	Acyclovir	P, S, T	Tablet 200 mg, 400 mg, 800 mg; Powder for injection 250 mg, 500 mg; Oral liquid 400 mg/5 mL (p)
6.6.2: Anti-cytomegalovirus (CMV) medicines			
6.6.2.1	Valganciclovir	S, T	Tablet 450 mg; Powder for oral solution 50 mg/mL
6.7: Medicines used in the Management of HIV			
6.7.1: Nucleoside Reverse Transcriptase Inhibitors			
6.7.1.1	Abacavir	S, T	Tablet 60 mg (p), 300 mg
6.7.1.2	Abacavir (A) + Lamivudine (B)	S, T	Tablet 60 mg (A) + 30 mg (B) (p), 600 mg (A) + 300 mg (B)
6.7.1.3	Lamivudine	S, T	Tablet 100 mg, 150 mg
6.7.1.4	Tenofovir Disproxil Fumarate (TDF)	S, T	Tablet 300 mg
6.7.1.5	Tenofovir Disproxil Fumarate (A) + Lamivudine (B)	S, T	Tablet 300 mg (A) + 300 mg (B)
6.7.1.6	Tenofovir Disproxil Fumarate (A) + Lamivudine (B) + Dolutegravir (C)	P, S, T	Tablet 300 mg (A) + 300 mg (B) + 50 mg (C)
6.7.1.7	Tenofovir Disproxil Fumarate (A) + Lamivudine (B) + Efavirenz (C)	S, T	Tablet 300 mg (A) + 300 mg (B) + 600 mg (C)
6.7.1.8	Zidovudine	S, T	Tablet 300 mg; Oral liquid 50 mg/5 mL (p)
6.7.1.9	Zidovudine (A) + Lamivudine (B)	S, T	Tablet 60 mg (A) + 30 mg (B) (p), 300 mg (A) + 150 mg (B)
6.7.1.10	Zidovudine (A) + Lamivudine (B) + Nevirapine (C)	S, T	Tablet 60 mg (A) + 30 mg (B) + 50 mg (C) (p), 300 mg (A) + 150 mg (B) + 200 mg (C)
6.7.2: Non-nucleoside Reverse Transcriptase Inhibitors			
6.7.2.1	Efavirenz	S, T	Tablet 200 mg (p), 600 mg
6.7.2.2	Nevirapine	P, S, T	Tablet 200 mg; Dispersible Tablet 50 mg (p); Oral liquid 50 mg/5 mL (p)
6.7.3: Integrase Inhibitors			
6.7.3.1	Dolutegravir	S, T	Tablet 50 mg
6.7.3.2	Raltegravir	S, T	Tablet 400 mg
6.7.4: Protease Inhibitors			
6.7.4.1	Atazanavir (A) + Ritonavir (B)	S, T	Tablet 300 mg (A) + Tablet 100 mg (B)
6.7.4.2	Darunavir	S, T	Tablet 600 mg
6.7.4.3	Darunavir (A) + Ritonavir (B)	S, T	Tablet 600 mg (A) + Tablet 100 mg (B)
6.7.4.4	Lopinavir (A) + Ritonavir (B)	S, T	Tablet 100 mg (A) + 25 mg (B), Tablet 200 mg (A) + 50 mg (B), Oral liquid 80 mg (A) + 20 mg (B)/mL (p); Capsule/Sachet (containing pellets/granules) 40 mg (A) + 10 mg (B) (p)
6.7.4.5	Ritonavir	S, T	Tablet 100 mg

	Medicine	Level of healthcare	Dosage form(s) and strength(s)
6.7.5: Medicines for Treating Opportunistic Infections in People Living with HIV			
6.7.5.1	Acyclovir	P, S, T	Injection 250 mg
6.7.5.2	Cefotaxime	P, S, T	Injection 1000 mg
6.7.5.3	Clindamycin	P, S, T	Tablet 300 mg
6.7.5.4	Clotrimazole	P, S, T	Ointment 1%
6.7.5.5	Valganciclovir	S, T	Tablet/Capsule 450 mg
6.7.6: Additional Medicines for Syndromic Management of Sexually Transmitted Infections			
6.7.6.1	Azithromycin	P, S, T	Tablet 1000 mg
Section 6.8: Medicines used in Hepatitis B and Hepatitis C			
6.8.1	Daclatasvir	S, T	Tablet 30 mg, 60 mg
6.8.2	Entecavir	S, T	Tablet 0.5 mg, 1 mg, Oral liquid 0.05 mg/mL (p)
6.8.3	Ribavirin	S, T	Capsule 200 mg
6.8.4	Sofosbuvir	S, T	Tablet 400 mg
6.8.5	Tenofovir alafenamide fumarate (TAF)	S, T	Tablet 25 mg
6.8.6	Tenofovir Disproxil Fumarate (TDF)	S, T	Tablet 300 mg
Section 6.9: Antiprotozoal Medicines			
6.9.1: Medicines for Amoebiasis and Other Parasitic Infections			
6.9.1.1	Metronidazole	P, S, T	Tablet 200 mg, 400 mg; Injection 500 mg/100 mL; Oral liquid 200 mg/5 mL (p)
6.9.2: Antileishmaniasis Medicines			
6.9.2.1	Amphotericin B	S, T	Amphotericin B (conventional): Injection 50 mg Lipid amphotericin B: Injection 50 mg Liposomal amphotericin B: Injection 50 mg
6.9.2.2	Miltefosine	P, S, T	Capsule 50 mg
6.9.2.3	Paromomycin	P, S, T	Injection 375 mg/mL
6.9.3: Antipneumocystosis and Antitoxoplasmosis Medicines			
6.9.3.1	Clindamycin	P, S, T	Capsule 150 mg, 300 mg
6.9.3.2	Co-trimoxazole [Sulphamethoxazole (A) + Trimethoprim (B)]	P, S, T	Tablet 400 mg (A) + 80 mg (B), Tablet 800 mg (A) + 160 mg (B), Oral liquid 200 mg (A) + 40 mg (B)/5 mL (p)
6.10: Antimalarial Medicines			
6.10.1: For curative treatment			
6.10.1.1	Artemether (A) + Lumefantrine (B)	P, S, T	Tablet 20 mg (A) + 120 mg (B), Tablet 40 mg (A) + 240 mg (B), Tablet 80 mg (A) + 480 mg (B)
6.10.1.2	Artesunate	P, S, T	Powder for injection 60 mg, 120 mg
6.10.1.3	Artesunate (A) + Sulphadoxine - Pyrimethamine (B)	P, S, T	Combi pack (A+B) 1 Tablet 25 mg (A) + 1 Tablet (250 mg + 12.5 mg)(B) 1 Tablet 50 mg (A) +1 Tablet (500 mg + 25 mg) (B) 1 Tablet 100 mg (A) + 1 Tablet (750 mg + 37.5 mg) (B) 1 Tablet 150 mg (A) + 2 Tablet (500 mg + 25 mg) (B) 1 Tablet 200 mg (A) + 2 Tablet (750 mg + 37.5 mg) (B)
6.10.1.4	Chloroquine	P, S, T	Tablet 150 mg; Oral liquid 50 mg/5 mL

	Medicine	Level of healthcare	Dosage form(s) and strength(s)
6.10.1.5	Clindamycin	P, S, T	Capsule 150 mg, 300 mg
6.10.1.6	Primaquine	P, S, T	Tablet 2.5 mg, 7.5 mg,15 mg
6.10.1.7	Quinine	P, S, T	Tablet 300 mg; Injection 300 mg/mL
6.10.2: For prophylaxis			
6.10.2.1	Doxycycline#	P, S, T	Capsule 100 mg; Oral liquid 50 mg/5 mL #for prophylaxis of *P. vivax*
6.10.2.2	Mefloquine#	T	Tablet 250 mg #Only for use as chemoprophylaxis for long-term travelers like military and travel troops, traveling from low endemic to high endemic area
Section 7: Anticancer Agents including Immunosuppressives and Medicines used in Palliative Care			
7.1: Antineoplastic Medicines			
7.1.1	5-fluorouracil	T	Injection 250 mg/5 mL
7.1.2	6-mercaptopurine	T	Tablet 50 mg
7.1.3	Actinomycin D	T	Powder for injection 0.5 mg
7.1.4	All-trans retinoic acid	T	Capsule 10 mg
7.1.5	Arsenic trioxide	T	Injection 1 mg/mL
7.1.6	Bendamusti ne hydrochloride	T	Injection 25 mg/vial; 100 mg/vial
7.1.7	Bleomycin	T	Powder for Injection 15 units
7.1.8	Bortezomib	T	Powder for Injection 2 mg
7.1.9	Calcium folinate	T	Tablet 15 mg; Injection 3 mg/mL
7.1.10	Capecitabine	T	Tablet 500 mg
7.1.11	Carboplatin	T	Injection 10 mg/mL
7.1.12	Chlorambucil	T	Tablet 2 mg, 5 mg
7.1.13	Cisplatin	T	Injection 1 mg/mL
7.1.14	Cyclophosphamide	T	Tablet 50 mg; Powder for Injection 500 mg
7.1.15	Cytosine arabinoside	T	Injection 100 mg/vial, 500 mg/vial,1000 mg/vial
7.1.16	Dacarbazine	T	Powder for Injection 200 mg Powder for Injection 500 mg
7.1.17	Daunorubicin	T	Injection 5 mg/mL
7.1.18	Docetaxel	T	Powder for Injection 20 mg, 80 mg
7.1.19	Doxorubicin	T	Injection 2 mg/mL
7.1.20	Etoposide	T	Capsule 50 mg; Injection 20 mg/mL
7.1.21	Gefitinib	T	Tablet 250 mg
7.1.22	Gemcitabine	T	Powder for Injection 200 mg, 1000 mg
7.1.23	Hydroxyurea	T	Capsule 500 mg
7.1.24	Ifosfamide	T	Powder for Injection 1000 mg, 2000 mg
7.1.25	Imatinib	T	Tablet 100 mg, 400 mg
7.1.26	Irinotecan HCl trihydrate	T	Solution for injection 20 mg/mL
7.1.27	L-asparaginase	T	Powder for Injection 5000 KU, 10000 KU
7.1.28	Lenalidomide	T	Capsule 5 mg, 25 mg
7.1.29	Melphalan	T	Tablet 2 mg, 5 mg

	Medicine	*Level of healthcare*	*Dosage form(s) and strength(s)*
7.1.30	Methotrexate	S, T	Tablet 2.5 mg, Tablet 5 mg, 10 mg; Injection 50 mg/mL
7.1.31	Oxaliplatin	T	Injection 5 mg/mL in 10 mL vial, 5 mg/mL in 20 mL vial
7.1.32	Paclitaxel	T	Injection 30 mg/5 mL,100 mg/16.7 mL
7.1.33	Rituximab	T	Injection 10 mg/mL
7.1.34	Temozolomide	T	Capsule 20 mg, 100 mg, 250 mg
7.1.35	Thalidomide	T	Capsule 50 mg, 100 mg
7.1.36	Trastuzumab	T	Injection 440 mg/50 mL
7.1.37	Vinblastine	T	Injection 1 mg/mL
7.1.38	Vincristine	T	Injection 1 mg/mL
7.2: Hormones and Antihormones used in Cancer Therapy			
7.2.1	Bicalutamide	T	Tablet 50 mg
7.2.2	Letrozole	T	Tablet 2.5 mg
7.2.3	Leuprolide acetate	T	Powder for injection 3.75 mg,11.25 mg, 22.5 mg
7.2.4	Prednisolone	S, T	Tablet 10 mg, 20 mg, 40 mg; Oral liquid 5 mg/5 mL (p), 15 mg/5 mL (p); Injection 20 mg/2 mL
7.2.5	Tamoxifen	T	Tablet 10 mg, 20 mg
7.3: Immunosuppressive Medicines			
7.3.1	Azathioprine	T	Tablet 50 mg
7.3.2	Cyclosporine	T	Capsule 25 mg, 50 mg,100 mg; Oral liquid 100 mg/mL (p); Injection 50 mg/mL
7.3.3	Mycophenolate mofetil	T	Tablet 250 mg, 500 mg
7.3.4	Tacrolimus	T	Capsule 0.5 mg, 1 mg, 2 mg
7.4: Medicines used in Palliative Care			
7.4.1	Allopurinol	S, T	Tablet 100 mg
7.4.2	Amitriptyline	S, T	Tablet 10 mg, 25 mg
7.4.3	Dexamethasone	S, T	Tablet 0.5 mg, 4 mg; Injection 4 mg/mL
7.4.4	Diazepam	S, T	Tablet 2 mg, 5 mg; Injection 5 mg/mL
7.4.5	Filgrastim	T	Injection 300 µg
7.4.6	Fluoxetine	S, T	Capsule 20 mg
7.4.7	Haloperidol	S, T	Tablet 1.5 mg, 5 mg; Injection 5 mg/mL
7.4.8	Lactulose	S, T	Oral liquid 10 g/15 mL
7.4.9	Loperamide	S, T	Tablet 2 mg
7.4.10	Metoclopramide	S, T	Tablet 10 mg; Oral liquid 5 mg/5 mL (p); Injection 5 mg/mL
7.4.11	Mesna	T	Injection 100 mg/mL
7.4.12	Midazolam	S, T	Injection 1 mg/mL
7.4.13	Morphine	S, T	Tablet 10 mg, Modified release tablet 30 mg
7.4.14	Ondansetron	S, T	Tablet 4 mg, 8 mg; Oral liquid 2 mg/5 mL (p); Injection 2 mg/mL
7.4.15	Tramadol	S, T	Capsule 50 mg, Capsule 100 mg; Injection 50 mg/mL
7.4.16	Zoledronic acid	T	Powder for injection 4 mg

	Medicine	Level of healthcare	Dosage form(s) and strength(s)
			Section 8: Medicines affecting Blood
8.1: Antianemia Medicines			
8.1.1	Erythropoietin	S, T	Injection 2000 IU/mL, 10000 IU/mL
8.1.2	Ferrous salts • Iron dextran • Iron sorbitol citrate complex	P, S, T	Tablet equivalent to 60 mg of elemental iron Injection 50 mg/mL, 50 mg/mL
8.1.3	Ferrous Salt (A)+ Folic acid (B)	P, S, T	Tablet 45 mg elemental iron (A) + 400 µg (B) Tablet 100 mg elemental iron (A) + 500 µg (B) Oral liquid 20 mg elemental iron (A) + 100 µg/mL (B) (p)
8.1.4	Folic acid	P, S, T	Tablet 1 mg, 5 mg
8.1.5	Hydroxocobalamin	P, S, T	Injection 1 mg/mL
8.1.6	Hydroxyurea	S, T	Capsule 500 mg
8.1.7	Iron sucrose	S, T	Injection 20 mg/mL
8.2: Medicines affecting Coagulation			
8.2.1	Enoxaparin	S, T	Injection 40 mg/0.4 mL, 60 mg/0.6 mL
8.2.2	Heparin	S, T	Injection 1000 IU/mL, 5000 IU/mL
8.2.3	Phytomenadione (Vitamin K_1)	P, S, T	Tablet 10 mg; Injection 10 mg/mL
8.2.4	Protamine Sulfate	S, T	Injection 10 mg/mL
8.2.5	Tranexamic acid	P, S, T	Tablet 500 mg; Injection 100 mg/mL
8.2.6	Warfarin	S, T	Tablet 1 mg, 2 mg, 3 mg, 5 mg
			Section 9: Blood Products and Plasma Substitutes
9.1: Blood and Blood Components			
9.1.1	Fresh frozen plasma	S, T	As licensed
9.1.2	Platelet rich plasma/platelet concentrates	S, T	As licensed
9.1.3	Red blood cells/packed RBCs	S, T	As licensed
9.1.4	Whole blood	S, T	As licensed
9.2: Plasma Substitutes			
9.2.1	Dextran-40	S, T	Injection 10%
9.3: Plasma Fractions for Specific Use			
9.3.1	Coagulation factor IX	S, T	Powder for injection 600 IU
9.3.2	Coagulation factor VIII	S, T	Powder for injection 250 IU, 500 IU
9.3.3	Cryoprecipitate	S, T	As licensed
			Section 10: Cardiovascular Medicines
10.1: Medicines used in Angina			
10.1.1	Diltiazem	P, S, T	Tablet 30 mg, 60 mg Modified release tablet 180 mg
		S, T	Injection 5 mg/mL
10.1.2	Glyceryl trinitrate	P, S, T	Sublingual tablet 0.5 mg
		S, T	Injection 5 mg/mL
10.1.3	Isosorbide dinitrate	P, S, T	Tablet 5 mg, 10 mg

	Medicine	Level of healthcare	Dosage form(s) and strength(s)
10.1.4	Metoprolol	P, S, T	Tablet 25 mg, 50 mg, 100 mg Modified release tablet 100 mg
		S, T	Injection 1 mg/mL
10.2: Antiarrhythmic Medicines			
10.2.1	Adenosine	S, T	Injection 3 mg/mL
10.2.2	Amiodarone	S, T	Tablet 100 mg, 200 mg; Injection 50 mg/mL
10.2.3	Digoxin	S, T	Tablet 0.25 mg; Oral liquid 0.05 mg/mL; Injection 0.25 mg/mL
10.2.4	Esmolol	S, T	Injection 10 mg/mL
10.2.5	Lignocaine	S, T	Injection 2%
10.2.6	Verapamil	S, T	Tablet 40 mg, 80 mg; Injection 2.5 mg/mL
10.3: Antihypertensive Medicines			
10.3.1	Amlodipine	P, S, T	Tablet 2.5 mg, 5 mg, 10 mg
10.3.2	Enalapril	P, S, T	Tablet 2.5 mg, 5 mg
10.3.3	Hydrochlorothiazide	P, S, T	Tablet 12.5 mg, 25 mg
10.3.4	Labetalol	P, S, T	Tablet 50 mg, 100 mg
		P, S, T	Injection 5 mg/mL
10.3.5	Ramipril	P, S, T	Tablet 2.5 mg, 5 mg
10.3.6	Sodium nitroprusside	S, T	Injection 10 mg/mL
10.3.7	Telmisartan	P, S, T	Tablet 20 mg, 40 mg, 80 mg
10.4: Medicines used in Shock and Heart Failure			
10.4.1	Digoxin	S, T	Tablet 0.25 mg; Oral liquid 0.05 mg/mL; Injection 0.25 mg/mL
10.4.2	Dobutamine	S, T	Injection 50 mg/mL
10.4.3	Dopamine	S, T	Injection 40 mg/mL
10.4.4	Noradrenaline	S, T	Injection 2 mg/mL
10.4.5	Spironolactone	P, S, T	Tablet 25 mg, 50 mg
10.5: Antiplatelet and Antithrombotic Medicines			
10.5.1	Acetylsalicylic acid	P, S, T	Conventional/Effervescent/Dispersible/Enteric coated Tablets 150 mg Conventional/Effervescent/Dispersible/Enteric coated Tablets 325 mg Enteric coated Tablet 75 mg Enteric coated Tablet 100 mg
10.5.2	Clopidogrel	P, S, T	Tablet 75 mg, 150 mg
10.5.3	Dabigatran	S, T	Tablet 110 mg, 150 mg
10.5.4	Enoxaparin	S, T	Injection 40 mg/0.4 mL, 60 mg/0.6 mL
10.5.5	Heparin	S, T	Injection 1000 IU/mL, 5000 IU/mL
10.5.6	Streptokinase	S, T	Injection 750, 000 IU, 15, 00, 000 IU
10.5.7	Tenecteplase	S, T	Injection 30 mg/vial, Injection 40 mg/vial
10.6: Hypolipidemic Medicines			
10.6.1	Atorvastatin	P, S, T	Tablet 10 mg, 20 mg, 40 mg, 80 mg
Section 11: Dermatological Medicines (Topical)			
11.1: Antifungal Medicines			
11.1.1	Clotrimazole	P, S, T	Cream 1%, Lotion 1%

	Medicine	Level of healthcare	Dosage form(s) and strength(s)
11.2: Antibacterial Medicines			
11.2.1	Framycetin	P, S, T	Cream 1%
11.2.2	Fusidic acid	P, S, T	Cream 2%
11.2.3	Silver sulphadiazine	P, S, T	Cream 1%
11.3: Antiinflammatory and Antipruritic Medicines			
11.3.1	Betamethasone valerate	P, S, T	Cream 0.05%, 0.1%
11.3.2	Calamine	P, S, T	Lotion (As per IP)
11.4: Keratolytic agents			
11.4.1	Benzoyl peroxide	P, S, T	Gel 2.5– 5%
11.4.2	Coal tar (A) + Salicylic Acid (B)	P, S, T	Solution 1% (A) + 3% (B)
11.4.3	Podophyllin resin	S, T	Solution 20%
11.4.4	Salicylic acid	P, S, T	Ointment 3–6%
11.5: Scabicides and Pediculicides			
11.5.1	Permethrin	P, S, T	Lotion 1%, Cream 5%
11.6: Miscellaneous			
11.6.1	Glycerin/glycerol (as mentioned in IP)	P, S, T	Topical
Section 12: Diagnostic Agents			
12.1: Ophthalmic Medicines			
12.1.1	Fluorescein	S, T	Ophthalmic strips
12.1.2	Proparacaine	S, T	Eye drops 0.5%
12.1.3	Tropicamide	S, T	Eye drop 1%
12.2: Radiocontrast Media			
12.2.1	Barium sulfate	S, T	Oral liquid 95% w/v
12.2.2	Gadobenate dimeglumine	T	Injection 529 mg/mL
12.2.3	Iohexol	S, T	Injection 140 to 350 mg iodine/mL
12.2.4	Meglumine diatrizoate	S, T	Injection 60% w/v, 76% w/v
Section 13: Dialysis Components (Hemodialysis and Peritoneal Dialysis)			
13.1	Haemodialysis fluid	S, T	As licensed
13.2	Peritoneal dialysis solution	S, T	As licensed
Section 14: Antiseptics and Disinfectants			
14.1: Antiseptics			
14.1.1	Chlorhexidine	P, S, T	Solution 5% (concentrate)
14.1.2	Ethyl alcohol (denatured)	P, S, T	Solution 70%
14.1.3	Hydrogen peroxide	P, S, T	Solution 6%
14.1.4	Methylrosanilinium chloride (gentian violet)	P, S, T	Topical preparation 0.25–2%
14.1.5	Povidone iodine	P, S, T	Solution 4–10%
14.2: Disinfectants			
14.2.1	Glutaraldehyde	S, T	As licensed
14.2.2	Potassium permanganate	P, S, T	Crystals for topical solution

	Medicine	*Level of healthcare*	*Dosage form(s) and strength(s)*
Section 15: Diuretics			
15.1	Furosemide	P, S, T	Tablet 40 mg; Oral liquid 10 mg/mL; Injection 10 mg/mL
15.2	Hydrochlorothiazide	P, S, T	Tablet 25 mg, 50 mg
15.3	Mannitol	P, S, T	Injection 10%, 20%
15.4	Spironolactone	P, S, T	Tablet 25 mg, 50 mg
Section 16: Ear, Nose and Throat Medicines			
16.1	Budesonide	P, S, T	Nasal spray 50 µg/dose, 100 µg/dose
16.2	Ciprofloxacin	P, S, T	Drops 0.3%
16.3	Clotrimazole	P, S, T	Drops 1%
16.4	Xylometazoline	P, S, T	Nasal drops 0.05%, 0.1%
Section 17: Gastrointestinal Medicines			
17.1: Antiulcer Medicines			
17.1.1	Omeprazole	P, S, T	Capsule 10 mg, 20 mg, 40 mg; Powder for oral liquid 20 mg
17.1.2	Pantoprazole	S, T	Injection 40 mg
17.2: Antiemetics			
17.2.1	Domperidone	P, S, T	Tablet 10 mg; Oral liquid 1 mg/mL
17.2.2	Metoclopramide	P, S, T	Tablet 10 mg; Injection 5 mg/mL
17.2.3	Ondansetron	S, T	Tablet 4 mg; Oral Liquid 2 mg/5 mL (p); Injection 2 mg/mL
17.3: Anti-inflammatory Medicines			
17.3.1	5- aminosalicylic acid (Mesalazine/Mesalaine)	S, T	Tablet 400 mg; Suppository 500 mg; Retention enema
17.4: Antispasmodic Medicines			
17.4.1	Dicyclomine	P, S, T	Tablet 10 mg; Oral solution 10 mg/5 mL; Injection 10 mg/mL
17.4.2	Hyoscine butyl bromide	P, S, T	Tablet 100 mg; Injection 20 mg/mL
17.5: Laxatives			
17.5.1	Bisacodyl	P, S, T	Tablet 5 mg; Suppository 5 mg
17.5.2	Ispaghula	P, S, T	Granules/Husk/Powder
17.5.3	Lactulose	S, T	Oral liquid 10 g/15 mL
17.6: Medicines used in Diarrhea			
17.6.1	Oral rehydration salts	P, S, T	As licensed
17.6.2	Zinc sulfate	P, S, T	Dispersible tablet 20 mg
17.7: Other Medicines			
17.7.1	Somatostatin	T	Powder for injection 3 mg
Section 18: Hormones, other Endocrine Medicines and Contraceptives			
18.1: Adrenal Hormones and Synthetic Substitutes			
18.1.1	Dexamethasone	S, T	Tablet 0.5 mg; Injection 4 mg/mL
18.1.2	Fludrocortisone	S, T	Tablet 0.1 mg
18.1.3	Hydrocortisone	P, S, T	Tablet 5 mg, 10 mg, 20 mg; Powder for injection 100 mg
18.1.4	Methylprednisolone	S, T	Injection 40 mg/mL
18.1.5	Prednisolone	P, S, T	Tablet 5 mg, 10 mg, 20 mg; Oral liquid 5 mg/5 mL (p), 15 mg/5 mL (p)

	Medicine	*Level of healthcare*	*Dosage form(s) and strength(s)*
18.2: Contraceptives			
18.2.1: Hormonal contraceptives			
18.2.1.1	Ethinylestradiol (A)+ Levonorgestrel (B)	P, S, T	Tablet 0.03 mg (A) + Tablet 0.15 mg (B)
18.2.1.2	Levonorgestrel	P, S, T	Tablet 0.75 mg, 1.5 mg
18.2.1.3	Ormeloxifene (Centchroman)	P, S, T	Tablet 30 mg
18.2.2: Intrauterine devices			
18.2.2.1	Hormone-releasing IUD	T	Contains 52 mg of Levonorgestrel
18.2.2.2	IUD-containing copper	P, S, T	As licensed
18.2.3: Barrier methods			
18.2.3.1	Condom	P, S, T	As licensed as per the standards of Drugs Rules, 1945
18.3: Medicines used in Diabetes Mellitus			
18.3.1: Insulins and other antidiabetic agents			
18.3.1.1	Glimepiride	P, S, T	Tablet 1 mg, 2 mg
18.3.1.2	Insulin (soluble)	P, S, T	Injection 40 IU/mL
18.3.1.3	Insulin intermediate acting (NPH)	P, S, T	Injection 40 IU/mL
18.3.1.4	Insulin glargine	P, S, T	Injection 100 IU/mL
18.3.1.5	Insulin Premix Injection 30:70 (Regular : NPH)	P, S, T	Injection 40 IU/mL
18.3.1.6	Metformin	P, S, T	Tablet 500 mg, 1000 mg Modified release tablet 1000 mg
18.3.1.7	Teneligliptin	P, S, T	Tablet 20 mg
18.3.2: Medicines used to treat hypoglycemia			
18.3.2.1	Glucose	P, S, T	Injection 25%
18.4: Ovulation Inducers			
18.4.1	Clomiphene citrate	T	Tablet 50 mg, 100 mg
18.4.2	Human chorionic gonadotropin	S, T	Injection 2000 IU, 5000 IU, 10000 IU
18.5: Progestogens			
18.5.1	Medroxyprogesterone acetate	P, S, T	Tablet 5 mg, 10 mg; Injection 150 mg/mL
18.5.2	Norethisterone	P, S, T	Tablet 5 mg
18.6: Thyroid and Antithyroid Medicines			
18.6.1	Carbimazole	P, S, T	Tablet 5 mg, 10 mg, 20 mg
18.6.2	Levothyroxine	P, S, T	Tablet 12.5 μg to 150 μcg (several strengths are available in market such as 12.5, 25, 50, 62.5, 75, 88, 100, 112 μg. Therefore, it was considered to give a range of available strengths)
Section 19: Immunologicals			
19.1: Diagnostic Agents			
19.1.1	Tuberculin, purified protein derivative	P, S, T	As licensed

	Medicine	Level of healthcare	Dosage form(s) and strength(s)
19.2: Sera and Immunoglobulins (Liquid/Lyophilized)			
19.2.1	Anti-rabies immunoglobulin	P, S, T	As licensed
19.2.2	Anti-tetanus immunoglobulin	P, S, T	As licensed
19.2.3	Anti-D immunoglobulin	S, T	As licensed
19.2.4	Diphtheria antitoxin	P, S, T	As licensed
19.2.5	Hepatitis B immunoglobulin	S, T	As licensed
19.2.6	Human normal immunoglobulin	T	As licensed
19.2.7	Snake venom antiserum	P, S, T	Soluble/liquid polyvalent (as licensed) Lyophilized polyvalent (as licensed)
19.3: Vaccines			
For Universal Immunization			
19.3.1	BCG vaccine	P, S, T	As licensed
19.3.2	DPT+ Hib+ Hep B vaccine	P, S, T	As licensed
19.3.3	DPT vaccine	P, S, T	As licensed
19.3.4	Hepatitis B vaccine	P, S, T	As licensed
19.3.5	Japanese encephalitis vaccine	P, S, T	As licensed
19.3.6	Measles vaccine	P, S, T	As licensed
19.3.7	Oral poliomyelitis vaccine	P, S, T	As licensed
19.3.8	Rotavirus vaccine	P, S, T	As licensed
19.3.9	Tetanus toxoid	P, S, T	As licensed
19.4: For Specific Group of Individuals			
19.4.1	Rabies vaccine	P, S, T	As licensed
Section 20: Medicines for Neonatal Care			
20.1	Alprostadil	S, T	Injection 0.5 mg/mL
20.2	Caffeine	S, T	Oral liquid 20 mg/mL; Injection 20 mg/mL
20.3	Surfactant	S, T	Suspension for intratracheal instillation (as licensed)
Section 21: Ophthalmological Medicines			
21.1: Anti-infective Medicines			
21.1.1	Acyclovir	P, S, T	Ointment 3%
21.1.2	Ciprofloxacin	P, S, T	Drops 0.3%; Ointment 0.3%
21.1.3	Natamycin	P, S, T	Drops 5%
21.1.4	Povidone iodine	P, S, T	Drops 5%
21.2: Anti-inflammatory Medicine			
21.2.1	Prednisolone	P, S, T	Drops 1%
21.3: Local Anesthetic			
21.3.1	Proparacaine	P, S, T	Drops 0.5%
21.4: Miotics and Antiglaucoma Medicines			
21.4.1	Acetazolamide	P, S, T	Tablet 250 mg
21.4.2	Latanoprost	P, S, T	Drops 0.005%
21.4.3	Pilocarpine	P, S, T	Drops 2%, 4%

	Medicine	*Level of healthcare*	*Dosage form(s) and strength(s)*
21.4.4	Timolol	P, S, T	Drops 0.25%, 0.5%
21.5: Mydriatics			
21.5.1	Atropine	P, S, T	Drops 1%; Ointment 1%
21.5.2	Homatropine	P, S, T	Drops 2%
21.5.3	Phenylephrine	P, S, T	Drops 5%, 10%
21.5.4	Tropicamide	P, S, T	Drops 1%
21.6: Miscellaneous			
21.6.1	Carboxymethyl cellulose	P, S, T	Drops 0.5%, 1%
21.6.2	Hydroxypropyl methylcellulose	T	Injection 2%
Section 22: Oxytocics and Antioxytocics			
22.1: Oxytocics and Abortifacient			
22.1.1	Dinoprostone	S, T	Tablet 0.5 mg; Gel 0.5 mg
22.1.2	Methylergometrine	P, S, T	Tablet 0.125 mg; Injection 0.2 mg/mL
22.1.3	Mifepristone	P, S, T	Tablet 200 mg
22.1.4	Misoprostol	P, S, T	Tablet 100 μg, 200 μg
22.1.5	Oxytocin	P, S, T	Injection 5 IU/mL, 10 IU/mL
22.2: Medicines used in Preterm Labor			
22.2.1	Betamethasone	P, S, T	Injection 4 mg/mL
22.2.2	Nifedipine	S, T	Tablet 10 mg
Section 23: Medicines used in Treatment of Psychiatric Disorders			
23.1: Medicines used in Psychotic Disorders			
23.1.1	Clozapine	T	Tablet 25 mg, 50 mg, 100 mg
23.1.2	Fluphenazine	P, S, T	Injection 25 mg/mL
23.1.3	Haloperidol	S, T	Tablet 2 mg, Tablet 5 mg, 10 mg, 20 mg; Oral liquid 2 mg/5 mL; Injection 5 mg/mL
23.1.4	Risperidone	P, S, T	Tablet 1 mg, 2 mg, 4 mg; Oral liquid 1 mg/mL; Injection (long acting) 25 mg, 37.5 mg
23.2: Medicines used in Mood Disorders			
23.2.1: Medicines used in depressive disorders			
23.2.1.1	Amitriptyline	P, S, T	Tablet 10 mg, 25 mg, 50 mg, 75 mg
23.2.1.2	Escitalopram	P, S, T	Tablet 5 mg, 10 mg, 20 mg
23.2.1.3	Fluoxetine	P, S, T	Capsule 10 mg, 20 mg, 40 mg, 60 mg
23.2.2: Medicines used in bipolar disorders			
23.2.2.1	Lithium	S, T	Tablet 300 mg
23.2.2.2	Sodium valproate	P, S, T	Tablet 200 mg, 300 mg, 500 mg; Modified release tablet 300 mg, 500 mg
23.2.2.3	Carbamazepine	P, S, T	Tablet 100 mg,200 mg, 400 mg, Modified release tablet 200 mg, 400 mg; Oral liquid 100 mg/5 mL (p)
23.3: Medicines used in Generalized Anxiety and Sleep Disorders			
23.3.1	Clonazepam	P, S, T	Tablet 0.25 mg, 0.5 mg, 1 mg
23.3.2	Zolpidem	P, S, T	Tablet 5 mg, 10 mg

	Medicine	Level of healthcare	Dosage form(s) and strength(s)
23.4: Medicines used in Obsessive Compulsive Disorders and Panic Attacks			
23.4.1	Clomipramine	P, S, T	Capsule 10 mg, 25 mg, 75 mg
23.4.2	Fluoxetine	S, T	Capsule 10 mg, 20 mg, 40 mg 60 mg
23.5: Medicines used in Disorders due to Psychoactive Substance Abuse			
23.5.1	Buprenorphine	P, S, T	Tablet (sublingual) 0.4 mg
23.5.2	Buprenorphine (A) + Naloxone (B)	P, S, T	Tablet (sublingual) 0.4 mg (A) + 0.1 mg (B) Tablet (sublingual) 2 mg (A) + 0.5 mg (B)
23.5.3	Nicotine (for nicotine replacement therapy)	P, S, T	Oral dosage forms 2 mg, 4 mg
Section 24: Medicines Acting on the Respiratory Tract			
24.1: Antiasthmatic Medicines			
24.1.1	Budesonide	P, S, T	Inhalation (MDI/DPI) 100 μg/dose, 200 μg/dose; Respirator solution for use in nebulizer 0.5 mg/mL, 1 mg/mL
24.1.2	Budesonide (A) + Formoterol (B)	P, S, T	Inhalation (MDI/DPI) 100 μg (A) + 6 μg (B) Inhalation (MDI/DPI) 200 μg (A) + 6 μg (B) Inhalation (MDI/DPI) 400 μg (A) + 6 μg (B)
24.1.3	Hydrocortisone	P, S, T	Powder for injection 100 mg, 200 mg
24.1.4	Ipratropium	P, S, T	Inhalation (MDI/DPI) 20 μg/dose Respirator solution for use in nebulizer 250 μg/mL
24.1.5	Montelukast	S, T	Tablet 4 mg, 5 mg (including chewable tablets),10 mg
24.1.6	Salbutamol	P, S, T	Tablet 2 mg, Tablet 4 mg; Oral liquid 2 mg/5 mL Inhalation (MDI/DPI) 100 μg/dose Respirator solution (solution for nebulizer 5 mg/mL)
24.1.7	Tiotropium	P, S, T	Inhalation (MDI) 9 μg/dose, Inhalation (DPI) 18 μg/dose
Section 25: Solutions Correcting Water, Electrolyte Disturbances and Acid-base Disturbances			
25.1.1	Glucose	P, S, T	Injection 5%, 10%, 25%, 50%
25.1.2	Glucose(A) + Sodium chloride (B)	P, S, T	Injection 5% (A) + 0.9% (B)
25.1.3	Oral rehydration salts	P, S, T	As licensed
25.1.4	Potassium chloride	P, S, T	Oral liquid 500 mg/5 mL
		S, T	Injection 150 mg/mL
25.1.5	Ringer lactate	P, S, T	Injection (as per IP)
25.1.6	Sodium bicarbonate	P, S, T	Injection (as per IP)
25.1.7	Sodium chloride	P, S, T	Injection 0.9%
		S, T	Injection 3%
25.2: Miscellaneous			
25.2.1	Water for injection	P, S, T	Injection
Section 26: Vitamins and Minerals			
26.1	Ascorbic acid (Vitamin C)	P, S, T	Tablet 100 mg, Tablet 500 mg
26.2	Calcium carbonate	P, S, T	Tablet 625 mg (equivalent to elemental calcium 250 mg) Tablet 1250 mg (equivalent to elemental calcium 500 mg)
26.3	Calcium gluconate	P, S, T	Injection 100 mg/mL
26.4	Cholecalciferol	P, S, T	Solid oral dosage form 1000 IU, 60000 IU; Oral liquid 400 IU/mL

	Medicine	Level of healthcare	Dosage form(s) and strength(s)
26.5	Pyridoxine	P, S, T	Tablet 10 mg, 50 mg,100 mg
26.6	Riboflavin	P, S, T	Tablet 10 mg
26.7	Thiamine	P, S, T	Tablet 100 mg; Injection 100 mg/mL
26.8	Vitamin A	P, S, T	Capsule/Tablet 50000 IU (including Chewable Tablet), Oral liquid 100000 IU/mL; Injection 50000 IU/mL
Section 27: Medicines for COVID 19 management			
27.1	Dexamethasone	P, S, T	Tablet 0.5 mg, 2 mg, 4 mg; Oral liquid 0.5 mg/5 mL (p); Injection 4 mg/mL
27.2	Enoxaparin	S, T	Injection 40 mg/0.4 mL, 60 mg/0.6 mL
27.3	Methylprednisolone	S, T	Injection 40 mg/mL
27.4	Paracetamol	P, S, T	Tablet 500 mg, 650 mg; Oral liquid 120 mg/5 mL (p), 125 mg/5 mL (p), 250 mg/5 mL (p)
27.5	Oxygen	P, S, T	As licensed for medical purpose